D0932910

GOING THE DISTANCE

Caring for a Loved One
With Lewy Body Dementia

.

Also by Betsy Jordan

Dante and Me: A Journey (Young Adult)

GOING THE DISTANCE

Caring for a Loved One
With Lewy Body Dementia

Betsy Jordan

GeniusWork Publishing
Los Angeles, CA

Published by GeniusWork Publishing
www.geniusworkpublishing.com

Printed in the United States of America
Cover Design by Sakada

Library of Congress Control Number: 2016938182

Cataloging-in-Publication data is on file with the publisher

ISBN 978-0-9831393-7-9 (paperback)
ISBN 978-0-9831393-8-6 (ebk)
ISBN 978-0-9831393-9-3 (ebk)

To Pete
Who always filled my heart with love

TABLE OF CONTENTS

ACKNOWLEDGMENTS

Writing is similar to caregiving, in that it is easier to do when you know you are supported and loved. Therefore, there are many people to thank—for supporting me through Pete's illness and passing, and through the writing of this book.

First and foremost, I thank my family: Pete's daughters—Katherine and Susan, and their families, my children—Amy, Myla, Jim, and John, and their families, and my sister Judy. Additional thanks to my granddaughters Erin and Meg, who set up my book's website and Facebook Page.

I am also grateful for so many friends, including Irish Flynn, Bill Pate, "Sickie" (our swim coach Ron Marcikic), Pat and Gail–my fellow Dementia Wives, Ken Fousel, Geraldine, and all the swimmers who nourished Pete and me.

Additionally, I am filled with gratitude for Dr. Paul Speckart and the staff at the Coronado Retirement Village Memory Care Unit.

Thanks to Penny Wilkes, I had the assistance and support of a writing coach, Sakada. I am immensely grateful for Sakada's help and advice, and for Penny's original referral.

And last, but far from least, I would like to thank Bella. She was my caregiver, giving me the medicine of unconditional love. She is always glad to see me when I come home. She nestles her warm muzzle on me when I am reading in bed. She was my biggest plus factor in dealing with caregiver stress, and she has been my wonderful companion through the grief of losing Pete. I can't wait to read this book to her!

"Where there is love there is life."

Mahatma Gandhi

DO IT WITH LOVE

Caring for a loved one in need is all about going the distance. Caring for a loved one with Lewy Body Dementia makes the distance especially long.

I am a long distance swimmer so I know about distances. I know that I need to get in the water, make a commitment, pace myself, and bring infinite patience and perseverance to the swim. I also need to love what I am doing – even through choppy waves, relentless swells, and uncomfortably cold water. All of these things apply to caregiving.

This is my personal story, but I also hope to help other caregivers. What I most want to tell you is to do it with love. Caregiving can be one of the most difficult challenges you will face in your life. Just as in long distance swimming, love is the most important thing you can bring to the challenge. Remember, you need to make it through those choppy waves, relentless swells, and very cold water —you need love to do this.

Focusing on your caregiving as a mission of love will sustain and carry both you and your loved one through all the ups and downs. This means prioritizing love in all your caregiving actions and keeping love front-and-center in all your caregiving decisions.

I was lucky that my marriage to Pete before he was diagnosed was an extremely loving one. Knowing that you love your loved one without limitation will sustain you through the long "swim" of caregiving. Knowing that you love what you are doing for him will bring you through difficult times.

Note that this mission of love has to include you. To be the best caregiver, you must take care of and love yourself, and you must do this during the caregiving, not just after. No matter how great the needs of your loved one, you must also take even better care of yourself since you are taking on the very large role of caregiver.

THE DISTANCE

Get in the Water and Make a Commitment

Since Lewy Body Dementia is a neurological disease, you need to be involved as soon as possible. The disease is progressive, but does not always progress in a straight line. Therefore, you never know when it will affect your loved one. Your full involvement and commitment is needed from the beginning.

I will not soften the truth—this course will not be an easy one, but if you are going the distance, the first step is getting in the water and making a commitment.

Pace Yourself

Just like long distance swimming, caring for a loved one with LBD requires a large level of endurance. Therefore, pacing yourself is critical. When swimming a long distance swim race, you are much more likely to tire if your only focus is on the end of the swim. Instead, I focus my swim from buoy to buoy.

I also learned to create a "reservoir of love" during the easier times of caregiving. By being fully present to all of the love that was shared when Pete was cognitively "there" with me and feeling good, I created a reservoir from which to draw upon during the most challenging times.

Infinite Patience And Perseverance

Patience and perseverance are much easier to hold on

3

to when there is love. A person with a neurological disease like LBD has cognitive challenges as well as physical body symptoms, so caregiving requires a whole new level of patience. Alternatively, since LBD is not just a cognitive disease, and there are often physical complications such as weakening muscles, a caregiver needs to be able to persevere through some, at times, difficult and proactive caregiving.

CAREGIVING STAGES

While medical doctors and nurses may discuss stages of a disease with you, the stages I write about are for the caregiver. The first is denial. When you notice your loved one changing and possibly having trouble with a simple task or thought, you pass it off to "getting older." Later you wonder why you did not see the issue sooner, but you must forgive yourself quickly.

Next is the stage of realization. This should come with a truth-telling first visit to the doctor, maybe even without your loved one along. Once given a name, your loved one's condition becomes much more real. This is not easy, but it does allow you to move forward in positive ways. You can adjust your life to this new reality.

One day, the next marker on this journey makes itself known, and you realize that you can no longer care for your loved one at home. This is particularly significant when caregiving an LBD person.

Once the very difficult decision to put your loved one in a care home is made, there is still much to do. For one thing, explaining it to your loved one. Again, this is where the neurological issues of an LBD person complicate an already challenging situation.

Once in a care facility, the caregiving continues, but changes. While there is some relief because the entire day-to-day burden is no longer resting on your shoulders, there are also new things to deal with.

Finally, I have to include the final good-bye. What I did have in long distance swimming that I did not have in caregiving an LBD loved one was a clear path and a desire to get to the destination. Modern medicine does not provide much clarity, so the path is often unknown. On the other hand, whether one actively acknowledges it or not, the destination is known, but it is not a destination at which you want to arrive. You do not want to lose your loved one.

I will say that while I miss my dear husband Pete every day, I am also so glad that our long distance journey with LBD was begun and completed with love. Every stage was filled with love.

MY LOVE LETTER TO YOU

In many ways, this book is my love letter to you, the caregiver.

This book actually started when Pete was first diagnosed. My husband was well known and loved by many friends and family, so in order to keep all these people in the loop, I started a Fans of Pete e-mail to update them. Because of the encouragement of many who received those e-mails, I wrote this book.

I truly hope that this book, and my story, will help you understand and deal with your LBD loved ones, and yourself, as compassionately as possible. After all, the whole progression of the disease builds upon the relationship between those who need love and those who give love.

I wish I had had such a personal guidebook myself, to help me find the best route for this last "swim" with Pete. I hope that remembering my own emotions and worries, as well as suggesting strategies for navigating the inevitable pitfalls of LBD, can help other caregivers. In addition, I will tell you my stories, including both the ups and the downs.

I offer this book as a personal beacon for others caring for loved ones adrift in the often unfathomable world of Lewy Body Dementia.

~1~
THE TUESDAY AFTER LABOR DAY

He had agreed to be admitted to the hospital. We prepared for it the whole holiday weekend. We talked to his daughters by phone about it. We discussed it on the way to the hospital. But no one can really be prepared for something like this. I could feel his anxiety as he held onto my hand in the emergency room.

After about three hours in a small curtained room, an attendant came to take him for admission. As she wheeled him down the hall, the nurse told me I couldn't go with them. I could only watch from a distance.

His large body was awkward in the small wheelchair and when they were fifteen feet away, his head started to turn to the left, and then his body tried to shift. He looked back, his left arm outstretched, reaching toward me. He wanted to see me and I realized he couldn't.

I wanted to run to him but I was frozen to my spot. They needed to take him to his hospital room and the most loving thing that I could do at that point was to not make a scene, not make this harder.

But when he reached his left arm back toward me and I could tell from even a side view that his face had erupted into worry and fear, I was heartbroken that I couldn't go to him. His in-control Navy SEAL persona was cracking. I knew he was feeling afraid and lonely.

"What if he thinks I don't care?" stabbed into me. I had to keep reminding myself that what we were doing was the right thing to do, the best avenue for him.

Looking back, I would see this as the most heart-wrenching moment I would feel during the whole course of his illness. Even now this image remains with me, and fills me with grief and guilt.

The man in the wheelchair was my beloved husband Pete. We had been married nearly twenty years and he had always been my rock. He, the kind giant who embodied both gentlemanliness and extreme mental toughness—not to mention topnotch physical conditioning—was sliding down into an irreparable void. Now I needed to be the rock for him. I resolved to double my love and compassion.

At that point a new world opened up—a new world where I could no longer take care of Pete in our house. His Lewy Body Dementia was getting worse and nothing brought this home more harshly than having Pete taken to a care facility. It was a stunning point of realization, and it hurt deeply on many levels.

~ ~ ~

The waters had been incredibly calm and idyllic for Pete and me before his LBD diagnosis. We were blessed to find each other and to join in a new marriage—the second for both of us. We felt particularly fortunate that our children, his two girls and my two sons and two daughters, got along beautifully and cheered our marriage plans. We were kindred souls. We loved each other beyond measure.

We both loved our children, making their wellbeing, education, and care top priorities. As our families expanded, our love swelled to encompass sons-in-laws and grandchildren. Visiting them in faraway states was a frequent activity. Cheering them on in their athletic contests ranked high. We welcomed them whenever possible in our home and always in our hearts. We had a lovingly blended family. We had a blessed life.

But that was before Lewy Body Dementia.

~2~

WE'RE JUST
GETTING OLDER

There were signs long before Pete's diagnosis, but pinpointing the disease is tough, and I was naïve in the early stages.

"We're both in our late seventies, so of course we have memory and behavior quirks," I would tell myself. So although I had noticed some memory and behavior issues with Pete over the past several years, I did not pin them down to a serious illness. Much of what was happening could be ascribed to normal aging. I also told myself that Pete could have PTSD from his time in the military. After all, Pete served in the military and even volunteered to go back later in his life. He served active duty with the SEAL team in Vietnam in the mid-1960s, after several years working at a law firm.

My husband's mechanical and computational skills were not his strong suit, so having trouble with ATM machines, gas pumps, computers, and cell phones did not surprise me. "My husband was never able to master how to use some of those things!" I would say, not realizing that these were the signs that preceded the larger difficulties to come.

I even remember telling a friend, "His focus is rightly on more important matters—like his love for his children and grandchildren." To further "prove" I was right on this, I proceeded to tell this friend how concerned he was about people getting fair treatment in the courtroom and that that was why he had been such a great juvenile court judge. I realize now that my friend might have wondered why I would redirect my statement to a discussion about him being a judge, a topic that had nothing to do with her concern for my husband.

Yes, Pete's growing habit of repeating certain things was becoming noticeable. And yes, his "minor muddles" were accumulating. I began to wonder, and if I am honest here, a gnawing ache began to grow in my heart.

BAD GUYS

It also became more and more obvious that sleep was difficult for Pete. He often thought that "bad guys" were in the house.

It is true that we had had an intruder in our home at one point. Pete had heard a noise in the kitchen and actually saw the intruder, who took Pete's credit card from his wallet on the kitchen table, with the intent of going to the bank and getting money. Pete saw the burglar jump out of an open window and run away. After that incident, we made sure to lock the windows, strengthen the fence and install new outdoor locks.

Unfortunately, Pete became hyper-alert to the point of sleeping with a baseball bat on the floor next to his side of the bed. He wanted to "catch that guy." One night he phoned 911 five or six times, even though no intruders were evident. I began to wonder if his reactions were outside the range of normal concern, so I ramped up my nighttime awareness, sacrificing some of my own sleep in the process.

Meanwhile, Dr. Paul Speckart, our family physician and good friend, as well as the police who had answered the 911 calls, convinced him that it was better to keep one's cell phone next to the bed, instead of a baseball bat.

For Pete though, there were still bad guys out there. It was not uncommon for him to wake me in the middle of the night to show me the bad guy.

"Betsy, quick, quick. Come look." He gently but relentlessly tugged at my right shoulder. Once I finally sat up in bed, he pulled me to the window. We hugged the wall, while he cautioned me to hide behind the curtains so the bad guys wouldn't see us.

"There," he said with satisfaction. He was pointing at the house being constructed next door. "Do you see him, there on the roof?"

"No I don't see him," I would reply, hoping that my not seeing the bad guy would put the issue to rest. It did not.

"I need to find him," Pete said. Then he dropped my hand and left the bedroom. Before I took another breath, he was in the back yard. Since he had dragged me out of bed, I didn't even have a robe on, so I ran to the closet, grabbed a raincoat, and ran after my bad-guy-hunting husband.

I soon learned that denying the bad guys was not fruitful. Instead, I calmed him by telling him that he obviously scared the bad guy away. This made him feel better. He prided himself, as an ex-SEAL, in protecting others. I actually loved this about him. Still, protecting me from an imaginary intruder at 2 A.M. was not my cup of tea.

Eventually I could convince him to return to our bedroom. As we returned to sleep, I would spoon him, hugging his large, still muscular body close to mine, hoping that I could hold on to the Pete I knew, and pretending that everything was fine.

OTHER VIEWPOINTS

Meanwhile, if anyone suggested that Pete might be having a problem, I had seemingly logical answers. No one wants to go looking for trouble, and at that point in my life I did not even know about LBD.

Since I lived with him, I felt like I should be the first one to notice changes or symptoms. Now, I have come to realize that the people closest to the LBD person are sometimes blind to the first subtle changes. Sometimes those closest even miss the not-so-subtle changes.

I gradually revised my thinking and started to actually hear what others were saying. During a visit from Pete's older daughter Katherine, she told me that she was going to pick up her son from the airport herself rather than let him drive there to do it. She was worried about her father.

I started to tune in.

Pete had told her four times that he was going to pick up her son. She had dealt with a family member with a similar disease and had written about it, so she was attuned to noticing such changes.

Initially, I felt a little displaced by her insight, but I worked through my feelings and am thankful to this day that she told me about her concerns. I realized that I needed to pay more attention to Pete's behavior.

Others noticed changes in Pete too. Our swim coach, a friend of many years, began to speculate about Pete. He told me he wondered, since Pete repeated nonsensical statements or ignored helpful suggestions, when Pete might forget how to swim altogether. I initially laughed at that thought, but looking back, I see that it gave another slice of light to the truth that I was going to have to face.

Meanwhile Pete and our swim coach continued their ongoing repartee and jokes. Pete and his swimming friends kept up their familiar banter too. It often seemed he was still himself, with his self-deprecating wit and helpful nature. So, when things tipped back and forth between concern and calm, I was naive and trusting in choosing to focus on the calm. In those moments I could tell myself that the world seemed to be continuing as it always had been.

MORE SIGNS

Once, he was so agitated that he fell out of bed. The next day, I made sure there was a padded piece of carpet there.

He would often get up two or more hours early, get dressed, shaved, and ready to go to our regular 6 A.M. swim practice. I would explain to him that it was too early to go and that he should lie back down and rest. He would comply, but would lie wide awake on top of the covers, all dressed and ready.

Many of his unfounded worries were financial. "Will you photocopy the education plan updates and send them along to all the grandchildren? I want to make sure they know they can chart their own courses through school and college," he would ask me. Even though it was the seventh time he asked me this question that week, I could argue that it was a beautifully thoughtful and articulate request.

On the other hand, we both knew he had meticulously arranged for his grandchildren's education funds. Yet now his worries about it were relentless. He also worried about mortgage payments, health care insurance, and banking in general. I continued to be patient. Without raising my voice, I reassured him that all was well and thanked him for his careful planning.

I learned not to object to repeated questions and not to correct mistakes. Instead, I reassured Pete that all was well, and thanked him profusely for his careful planning and love for me, as well as for our children and grandchildren.

SORTING THIS OUT

As I mentioned, it is highly likely that Pete was dealing with the early symptoms of LBD for a considerable number of years before any of us began to recognize the symptoms. Looking back, I wish I had been more aware.

Ironically, it was Pete with whom I would have wanted to talk about all of this. But there were two reasons that talking to Pete was not a possibility: 1) he was the subject of the conversation, and 2) LBD was taking away his cognitive abilities and I could no longer completely trust his counsel.

This is one of the most difficult things about "losing" a loved one who is your partner, your shoulder to lean on, your counsel and confidant. Be it your spouse, your parent, or anyone with this role in your life, if your LBD loved one is someone you are accustomed to looking to for help, it is devastating to lose that person to this demon disease. Just when I needed his counsel most, he was not available to me. I would have asked Pete, "Do you think there is something more serious than 'old age' going on here?" Then I would have asked him, "What should we do?" And Pete would have come up with a solid plan and taken action. That was the kind of man he was.

But Pete was not consistently available, and with more and more responsibility falling on my shoulders, I began to feel overwhelmed. Of course, I also did everything I could to shield Pete from my worries. "You can do this," I told myself. But the worries took a toll on my sleep and my peace of mind.

~3~
DIAGNOSIS

Lewy Body Dementia is a complicated disease with both physical and cognitive symptoms, therefore presenting particular issues for physicians, patients, and caregivers. It is often misdiagnosed because the only absolutely positive diagnosis comes from an autopsy of the brain after death, identifying certain molecular configurations (Lewy bodies). The overlap with both Alzheimer's and Parkinson's diseases augments the confusion.

PETE'S FINAL 911 CALL

It was an early spring night, dark with no moonlight. I was dreaming. Pete and I were asleep in our king-size bed.

Something woke me. I looked at the bedside clock and it read 3:20 A.M. I heard a quiet speaking voice in the house. Suddenly, it hit me that a voice at that time of night was something to pay attention to. I opened my eyes and tried to tune into the voice, tried to hear what was being said.

Silence returned. The room was cool so I had pulled the covers up to my chin. I looked over to the other side of the bed–Pete wasn't there. "Maybe he has gotten up to go to the bathroom," I thought.

Then I heard the voice again, then more than one voice. Alarmed, I got out of bed and wrapped myself in a robe. Peeking into the living room, I saw a police car parked at the curb, lights flashing. Pete was talking with two policemen inside, but near the door. All three of them turned to look at me.

Seeing me, Pete said "Oh, she IS here."

Both of the policemen smiled.

I did not understand what was going on. I remembered how the two policemen and Pete were all of similar build. They filled the living room with their height and size.

One of the policemen said to me "He said you were missing."

20

The other policeman added, "He thought perhaps you had been abducted."

"No," I said, "I was sound asleep under the covers."

"Sit down," The first police officer walked me to the couch. Still confused, I thought that Pete must have had a bad dream. I didn't want to embarrass him, so I was quiet as the policemen wrote notes on their paper pads. I did tell them that we had had a break-in, as if that might provide some cover for Pete.

Now that I had joined the group, Pete became quiet. My heart was breaking for him. I realized that he had been quite vigorous in his original argument to the police that I had been abducted. Now that I was there, I could feel his confusion. He was caught between two realities, and it left him lost in the middle.

Here again, I saw my husband, sliding so deeply into his delusions, delusions that left him out of touch with reality. Yet, I also saw his brave heart, still thinking of me, still trying to protect me. The story in his head was made up, but it still made him my hero.

So I sat there, listening to the policemen talk, balancing my own confusion about what to do for Pete with a feeling of being overwhelmed. I think it was in that moment, while the police lights flashed and probably woke some neighbors, while Pete sat quietly and listened intently to the police officer's directions, while the sun crept closer to its rise, that I decided that whatever was in front of us,

I would take care of Pete and love him with all my heart. That is what I decided. That is what I did.

Before the policemen left, they said they would return in a few days with their staff psychologist. Pete bowed his head. I hugged him as we watched the policemen get into their cruiser and turn off their revolving red light.

They left. We locked the door and walked back into the bedroom. I could not even imagine what he was feeling. We got into bed and I put my arm around him. I didn't want him to think it was his fault. "Would you like a drink of water?" I asked as I moved closer to him so we could touch each other.

A few days later, two police officers visited. One of them was a staff psychologist. They suggested that Pete talk to his physician about the episode.

Pete was visibly embarrassed, but he covered it up well. "I am sorry for the inconvenience," he said, "I must have been mistaken." I could tell he was nervous having to say this to them, as if he had been "caught in the act," but he maintained his dignity. I was very proud of him.

The two policemen politely advised him not to be afraid of calling 911 again if something truly upsetting happened, but they also asked him to try to be "more precise about the difficulty" before calling again.

TIME TO GET INTO THE WATER

This event woke me up, literally and figuratively.

I realized that it was time to look at this more deeply. Up until now I was standing on the shore, and now it was time to truly enter the water and commit to Pete's care. I needed to take responsibility for him. I needed to love and care for him.

My Pete, the Pete I married, the Pete who had been my husband for nearly twenty years, was no longer there all the time. I also realized that I was beginning a marathon swim, not a sprint. For a marathon swim one needs careful preparation, pacing, and lots of courage. "You can do this," I told myself.

My head was filled with questions and concerns: How would I take care of Pete when he needed so much attention and care? How would I keep him safe? How would I calm his anxiety? How would I keep our home a safe and welcoming place for Pete? And how would I accommodate my own very real sadness?

DOCTOR VISITS
"My" Doctor's Appointment

It was also time to get help, professional help. The police had advised us to see our physician. Trying to give Pete the benefit of the doubt, I didn't call Dr. Speckart right away, but I did make an appointment for a month later. I wanted to talk to the doctor face to face—without Pete

For anyone facing early mental symptoms like this, talking with the family physician is a good starting point. Making the first appointment one between just you and your loved one's doctor is a good strategy.

Seeing your loved one's doctor on your own is also a difficult step. Pete and I had always shared everything. Together we made all our choices, and worked out all the concerns and issues we faced. Not only did I feel lonely in this decision, but I also wondered if I was betraying my husband. This was a big step for me, and I did not take it lightly.

But at this point I was in the swim and committed to Pete's care above all else. I had to put these worries aside. I arranged a time to talk with Dr. Speckart, and when Pete asked what I was doing that day, I just said I had a doctor's appointment. He wished me a good day!

Once I began talking to Dr. Speckart, I found out I had lots to share. "Here is what he is doing," I began. I started with the recent police call about my "abduction" and filled in with all my concerns and worries. Every now and then I felt like I was tattling on Pete, talking behind his back. I also knew I was doing this with love.

I have to admit, it was also a relief. I realized just how much worry I had been carrying, how much work it had been to hold everything together. Facing a loved one's illness is always about holding many things together, but when you are in the denial stage, you have to hold everything together including all your stories of denial. Denial is a heavy thing to hold.

It helped me to think in terms of a swim race. Pete and I both knew that instead of focusing on the finish line, using short term goals of completing the next stroke or the next turn, or going around the next buoy created more successful swims.

But I was now dealing with a life-changing health matter, not a simple race. In a swim race I would find joy at the completion, whether or not it was a victory. Here, in a severe illness, where would I find that joy? I was determined to seek it out–whenever and wherever possible.

Dr. Speckart recognized a brain disease immediately, and gave me some samples of dementia drugs. I took them home, but left them unused on a bathroom shelf. I was not ready to start giving Pete drugs until Pete himself was aware of his condition.

A month later, when Dr. Speckart spoke with both Pete and me, he relaxed Pete by talking with him about American history, which they both loved. He didn't specifically call Pete's situation dementia. But a few months later, when I again talked with Dr. Speckart alone, he labeled it Lewy Body Dementia. He recognized it because he had seen several patients with these symptoms. He recommended that I take Pete to see a neurologist.

Up to this point neither Dr. Speckart nor I had mentioned the word "dementia" to Pete. I feared what Pete's reaction to that word might be.

The Neurologist

"Why do I have to count backward from 100 by sevens?" Pete asked me, during the first visit with the neurologist.

His tall frame balanced awkwardly on the examination table while I watched from a chair.

The neurologist's test about memory—naming four things at the beginning of the appointment and then recalling them later—unnerved Pete. I could almost see his brain searching for answers as he tried to recall the items he had named earlier. The neurologist also tested Pete's balance and walking.

After all the "tests," I asked the neurologist if there was a specific name for Pete's condition. He told us that it was called MCI, or Mild Cognitive Impairment. So, at last a diagnosis expressed openly to Pete! He reacted calmly but later had lots of questions and comments.

I collected some information about MCI and read it out loud to Pete. I learned, and repeated to Pete, that MCI sometimes goes away or improves, but that it can also progress into dementia.

"If MCI sometimes goes away," Pete would say, "I don't need those drug samples Dr. Speckart gave you. I'll work at it and just get better on my own."

I took the drug samples back to Dr. Speckart's office.

Meanwhile, Pete decided to work on his memory issues with workbooks. He asked me to buy him some third grade level math books so he could improve his computing skills. His years at Yale, at the University of Chicago Law School, and in the military, had convinced him that just applying a little more elbow grease and a strong work ethic could and would improve his situation.

Furthermore, his mental toughness about thorough preparation, learned through school and work, was deep-rooted and he applied it in preparing for his neurology appointments.

Despite his preparation, he would still get fidgety and uneasy several days before the appointments. He couldn't concentrate on reading the newspapers or watching news or sports on television. He knew that the visits always included tests, and that idea terrified him.

When he realized he had difficulty counting backward from 100 by sevens, he asked me to practice with him over and over again. I kept reassuring him that doctors give tests because tests help them determine the best care for patients, but it was still nerve-wracking for him.

At the appointments, I watched him in the waiting room, unable to relax and look at a magazine. He was outwardly his usual personable self, chatting with everyone we encountered, the other patients, the nurses, and the neurologist, but the tension in his voice and manner revealed his anxiety to me.

"Let's go out for lunch after we see the doctor," I would offer, finding that combining a trip to the doctor with something else that was more fun was a great distraction strategy. Already I was straining my own abilities to deal with his challenges, but I explored all the avenues I could think of. A new plan of action or even a change of subject matter always seemed to help.

A NEW STAGE
A Diagnosis

Now we had a diagnosis. For Pete, the diagnosis of Mild Cognitive Impairment propelled him into action. It warmed my heart to see his determination to "beat" MCI. Of course, it did not surprise me. Pete was a man of action!

I was happy that the neurologist diagnosed Pete's condition as MCI, and told this to Pete, but the term "Lewy Body Dementia" still stuck in my head. I had researched both on the internet. So while MCI was our first buoy, I was still worried about LBD.

At this point the diagnosis was two-part. I knew more about it than Pete did. To me, Pete had MCI and also had LBD, according to Dr. Speckart. To Pete, he had only MCI, according to the neurologist. Neither Dr. Speckart nor I felt ready to put the extra burden of LBD on Pete's shoulders.

~ ~ ~

Seeing the neurologist instigated a new stage, and it had come with some big realizations.

The good news was that Pete and I could continue our life together in our own home. This felt great.

There were also lots of worries. Being on alert all the time takes its toll. Indeed, I was in the water and committed to taking care of Pete with love and compassion. I knew I had to pace myself. I also knew I was going to have to call on my patience in whole new ways. Perseverance would be key. But as soon as I took the first steps forward, I knew that I would somehow find the strength to take care of Pete, and to take care of myself.

Every night, I wrapped my arms around my husband and held him tight, remembering that this was a mission of love.

~4~
CAREGIVING AT HOME

"Betsy, I have to get up."

Difficulty sleeping and loss of muscle control are common with LBD patients. This meant many middle-of-the-night trips to the toilet. Since Pete was often groggy at night, he needed my help getting to and from the bathroom.

It is not easy to be roused out of a deep sleep and get yourself alert enough to help your loved one. I did though, feel as if I got better at these late night and early morning situations. For one thing, I got lot of practice.

Pete had really low blood pressure so I made sure he sat on the edge of the bed a few moments before standing up, to avoid fainting.

We would laugh about the giraffe syndrome—"You're six and a half feet tall. We need to get some blood to your brain before you get up!"

He would smile, and that smile would thrill me. Caregiving gives you so many small unexpected joys. To this day, looking back and remembering his smile about the giraffe syndrome is one of those joys.

Once he felt stable, I helped him stand and walk. He was a big man and I guided him one step at a time, putting my arm tightly around him. I learned to be peaceful and helpful, even when he would miss the target and urinate in the wastebasket or on the floor.

Despite having a waterproof cover on the mattress, on some nights, after he finished in the bathroom, I would take him to the living room.

"You rest here while I fix up the bed a little."

I would then dry the mattress with a hair dryer and put on clean sheets. I did a lot of laundry in the middle of the night. It was only when the bedroom was clean and ready that I would return to the living room, where he was usually asleep on the sofa. It would take another ten minutes to wake him enough to help him back to bed.

Then I would lie down next to him so we could touch each other, and tell him I loved him.

24/7
Quick Errands & Take-Alongs

Almost all our family members live out of state, so Pete was my responsibility, and somehow, I managed it. If you ask me now what I did, I don't know if I could tell you. But somehow, I found a way to take care of Pete and get things done.

At first I could leave Pete alone for short periods of time. For longer errands I would take Pete with me. At the grocery store, pushing the cart appealed to him. But sometimes I just needed to go alone.

Occasionally I left him at home while the person who helped me with housecleaning was there. But that was only a temporary solution because, after all, her job was to clean the house, not to worry about Pete or take responsibility for his actions.

Luckily beyond errands, we did most things together. In particular, he was still swimming, so I didn't have to give up my swimming or leave him alone.

Supervision

Eventually, Dr. Speckart cautioned me that Pete should not be left alone. There were just too many pitfalls, too many opportunities for situations that could be dangerous, and too many worries for me.

Realizing this made me incredibly sad but also gave me incentive to stay afloat. There are many moments like this in caregiving. They are extremely sad or challenging, but also illuminating, and can inspire you on your journey. One of the things that can be very useful to caregivers is the ability to turn a challenge into an opportunity to truly take care of your loved one – and to do it with lots of love.

Not leaving someone alone may sound simple enough, but it is actually extremely difficult. How do you do everything you need to do without leaving your loved one alone? Even something as routine as grocery shopping or a quick errand becomes problematic.

I tried hiring a helper to come to our home several times a week. Then a neighbor came to tell me that while I was out, Pete had walked across the street multiple times to knock at her door. It became clear that finding a helper with whom I felt comfortable was not going to be easy. I decided that hiring a helper, no matter how good, was never the same as being there to look out for Pete myself.

Even when I was home with Pete, the need to supervise him became more intense. Luckily, Pete was not as consistent in his wandering as some LBD patients, but I worried. For one thing, when looking for "bad guys," he would sometimes go out the back door or into the front yard to look for them. I feared that one day he would open the back gate, which leads to a busy street, so I followed him like a hawk.

I always wanted to put a good face on our situation, so that friends and neighbors wouldn't worry, either about him or about me. I was able to keep up this façade, but inside, to be honest, I was struggling more and more. Being on alert 24/7 is stressful. It was a good thing that this was a mission of love!

PETE'S HURTFUL DELUSIONS

In the early stages of home caregiving, I would leave Pete at home while I went to a local yoga class. One morning, in the middle of the class, I happened to look over toward the door. In the midst of doing a "downward dog" pose, I saw a tall man standing outside the door looking in.

"Oh my gosh, it's Pete!" I thought, but I said nothing.

He was searching the room with his eyes, trying to verify that I was really going to yoga class, as I said I was. The class was held very close to our home, so he could easily walk there.

Even though I knew he was there I continued to look straight ahead at the mirror, pretending I had not seen him He watched quietly for a few minutes and then went on his way, returning home.

I continued to concentrate on my yoga poses, but inside, I was in turmoil. No matter how much I understood it was an LBD delusion, it was still upsetting when he mistrusted me. Specifically, a recurring delusion that I had a boyfriend was taking shape and growing in his mind. Sometimes he even accused me of wanting to divorce him.

~ ~ ~

Pete's delusion that I had a boyfriend could show up at any time – and it always surprised me:

One day Pete and I had lunch with my sister Judy and some mutual friends. This was a great break for me. At this point I could not leave Pete alone at home, but with this group he was welcome to join in. In fact, Pete was the star of the event. He was happy. Not only was everyone focused on him and his stories, but he also got to feast on his favorite tuna sandwiches at our favorite seafood restaurant.

After lunch, because my car was a block away, I asked him to wait just inside the restaurant with my sister so he wouldn't have to walk to the car. She stayed with him until I pulled the car up to the front sidewalk.

Pete slid into the car and asked "So, were you calling your boyfriend on the cell phone?"

He never spoke angrily--anger had no place in his personality--but he was firm in his tone.

"Pete!" I felt deflated. This had been such a nice outing for us, but Pete's comment completely unnerved me.

"You were calling your boyfriend, weren't you?"

I took a moment to regroup and said, "Pete, I don't have a boyfriend. I'm married to you. Thank you for marrying me. I love you."

Until the person behind me honked, I didn't even realize that cars were piling up behind us while I tried to alleviate Pete's worry about an imaginary boyfriend. The honk made me turn my attention back to driving.

We didn't talk the rest of the way home. I used the time to settle down and calm my own hurt. I reminded myself that it was those brain gremlins that created this belief in Pete. I targeted my anger at the gremlins, which allowed me to forgive and love Pete.

Meanwhile, "my Pete" came back and said he knew I loved him.

This was true to the quick high/low emotional succession of LBD. He would accuse me of infidelity one minute, and quickly come right back, asserting how happy he was that we were married and how fortunate we were that we both loved each other as much as we did. I would breathe a sigh of relief but knew this would happen again. His worries would emerge, then subside, and then re-emerge. It is a cycle you must learn to accept with your LBD loved one.

This suspicious Pete wasn't the Pete who was my adored life partner. This was Pete with a brain disease. The dissociation between past and present, between health and disease, between delusion and reality, was here to stay.

I sometimes found myself sinking into an emotional pit about not having my old loving Pete with me as before. In the end, I would simply resolve to love him even more—like going an extra half mile in the ocean after I had already completed what I had set out for myself that day.

PHYSICAL CHALLENGES

Pete was a big man. The more he needed me to help him get up and walk, the more his size worried me. I'm a strong person but I am a year older than Pete and maybe sixty pounds lighter. Helping him at home in our own bedroom was one thing, but as the LBD progressed, Pete could get sleepy in all kinds of situations.

If I stopped for breakfast after swimming, he would often fall asleep in the car after we had eaten. As he became drowsy, his head would slump down on his chin and his shoulders would move to the left, toward the steering wheel. His hands would sometimes reach out toward the driver's side of the car, or worse, toward the door handles on the right. I worried about him leaning into the gearshift or reaching for the door while the car was moving. I also worried about how I would get Pete safely out of the car and into the house.

Eventually, I would focus our outings on one event at a time–either swimming or breakfast, not swimming and breakfast.

MORE CHANGES
Driving

We both had cars, but Pete had always been the principal driver. Before the "never leave him alone" rule, Pete continued to drive.

At first, with the diagnosis of MCI, we didn't even think about him not driving. But he could get easily confused about directions, so when he had an appointment somewhere in an area not well known to him, he would ask me for advice.

"How do I get to the bank from swim practice?" he would say.

I would write out directions, draw him a map, and tape it to the dashboard in his car.

A turning point occurred when he got lost driving to a doctor's appointment despite the written directions. Pete, known for punctuality and for always arriving early, had to tell the doctor that he had gotten lost.

Later he told me, with sadness in his voice, "The doctor pleaded with me not to drive any more."

I ached for Pete. I imagined how he must have felt when the doctor pressured him about this. Yet fortunately, the physician's plea triggered Pete's own decision to stop driving.

"I might hurt some little child," he said.

While I welcomed Pete's decision, I also worried

about how he would accept and process this decision. This is often the dilemma of the caregiver: how to balance good decisions with the effects of those decisions on your LBD loved one. With LBD, each step in seems to take something away from your loved one. And yet, it is love that allows you to make, and "enforce" such decisions.

We returned his car to the dealer where he was leasing it, and he never complained about his loss of freedom. "No whining" had long ago been instilled in him, in school and in the Navy.

His retirement from driving made my life much calmer. At the same time, I knew that having to ask me for transportation was a huge and limiting factor for him, and it meant that I was now accountable for all his transportation. This was an added responsibility for me, the caregiver.

Later, when I attended support groups for LBD, I found out what a daunting hurdle the "no driving" rule caused for other caregivers. I was fortunate that I didn't have to go to extremes to make sure he couldn't renew his driver's license. Some in the support group had stories about surreptitiously telling the DMV test-givers to make sure their loved ones didn't pass the test, or hiding the car keys. I never had to beg Pete not to drive.

Finances

After Pete stopped driving, I would drive him to the ATM machine at the bank and wait in the car for him while he withdrew cash. One morning, I watched him at the cash machine, but was also focused on other things, in my head and on the radio. So I did not realize right away that Pete had been at the ATM for over fifteen minutes. I knew he was just withdrawing cash.

When he showed me the receipts from the machine, it was clear that he needed multiple attempts to make a $200 withdrawal. First he would get $20 and then he would have to initiate a second request, then a third withdrawal. After three withdrawals he had $180.

My first reaction was impatience, but I soon realized he was doing his best. I also realized that these mechanical and mathematical procedures were slipping out of his grasp.

~~~

Several times a month, Pete and I would sit at the dining room table and work on paying bills. One day I noticed him writing $400 on a check when he meant $40, so I realized that more changes needed to be made. I suggested that I would write his checks and he could sign them, which he could do perfectly well. This solution did not seem unusual or difficult for him, and I was grateful and relieved.

As I learned later, many caregivers faced loved ones who were less compliant. I was blessed! But unlike before, I was now stepping into the "financial manager" role for us. More responsibility and more caregiving.

MAKING THE BEST OF IT
Swimming

Pete's swimming and walking slowed down, and he couldn't really run any more. Luckily, we still had our swimming. For one thing, swimming was a very healthy activity for Pete. It was also something that we shared. Both of us participated in Masters Swimming training and long distance ocean swimming. Finally, swimming can be a very social activity. We had long-time friends in all of our swimming activities. In fact, it was because of these friends that I could continue to take Pete to the University of California San Diego (UCSD) for our Master Swimming workouts. Our male friends helped Pete in the locker room.

I would meet Pete at the locker room door and together we would walk out to the pool deck and jump in, breaking up the water's surface into little bright splashes. Then we would hang on to the pool gutter, and look up, waiting to hear our assignment for the morning. Although from our vantage point we could only see the coach's shoes and socks, we knew he was smiling down on us and always had some upbeat remarks.

Since Pete and I had a tradition of kissing when we first entered the pool, our coach would laugh and say "No smooching!" Pete would smile and light up, being so pleased with himself, and I would be delighted too. I loved those beautiful moments of light when Pete and I and our coach were one.

Pete no longer understood the pace clock but that didn't matter. I swam in the lane with him and would just suggest to him that "Now we are doing freestyle" or whatever the assignment was.

After our swim, he would go back into the locker room with his friends. Fellow swimmers soon learned to help him with his clothing. As I waited for him outside the locker room his friends would emerge and give me smiling reports: "He's making progress, he has his left sock on!"

His friends also learned that Pete tended to misplace things, or to pick up things not belonging to him. Once a swim friend came running after us in the parking lot saying "I think Pete has my underwear in his swim bag!"

One of my biggest concerns was how he felt about himself, although he seemed blithely unaware of any problems. He seemed to feel quite at home with who he was. If he noticed how his friends were looking out for him in the locker room, he didn't mention it.

While his swimming buddies were nothing but generous and kind, I felt increasingly awkward about our situation. From being so competent before, Pete had metamorphosed into a forgetful and sometimes naïve man. For me, these changes loomed over us.

SPECIAL JOYS
Family

Friends and family are special joys in general, but during a caregiving situation, they truly sparkle.

Family is the best resource of all. Throughout his illness, Pete and I spent many hours looking through scrapbooks and photo albums. He also loved the frequent notes and calls from our children, and artwork from his grandchildren. A benefit of his weakening memory was that mementos could be re-enjoyed over and over again. He wouldn't remember that I had read a letter or shown him a drawing in the past, so each time I showed it to him, it was like a new treat.

Of course, Pete loved special occasions like Thanksgiving, when family members visited from far away. I would cook foods that he loved, while our children and grandchildren doted on him.

Friends

Pete's Navy friends really stepped up to the plate to help out, with continuing and unwavering kindness. One of Pete's favorite outings was when his friend, Irish Flynn, took him to the quarterly "Old Frogs" meetings. Pete felt so at home with his fellow SEALS. The dinners gave Pete the chance to share some of his old Navy stories to receptive audiences. Bless each and every one of you who listened to Pete, who laughed with him, who made him proud to be a SEAL.

Our swimming friends were also so supportive, both at the pool and the ocean. One example of this is a one-mile swim race in which Pete desperately wanted to participate. This was late summer in 2013, and I was worried about his physical ability to complete the race.

Pete insisted and entered the competition. I decided to stay on shore with the lifeguards, rather than swim with him. I felt as if I could better monitor Pete from the shore. Also, the water temperature had dropped to 57 degrees, which was too cold for me.

I quietly mentioned my fears to the race organizers, telling them that my husband Pete suffered from dementia and would be slow, so please look out for him. I knew his thinking was awry because just that morning he had asked me, when we were getting up and dressed in our home in Coronado, if we were in Chicago. Unbeknownst to him, the race organizers assigned one lifeguard on a paddleboard to stay alongside him.

Just before the race was to begin, our friends Geraldine and Richard arrived, wanting to enter. Richard got there in time to put in his entry fee, but Geraldine, who was still parking the car a few blocks down the street, got there too late to enter.

When I told her what Pete was doing, she noticed my panicky worries and said, "Well, I'll just swim next to him. I'll tell him I need his assistance since he knows this Coronado ocean better than I do. It doesn't matter that my swim will be unofficial."

The competitors were to swim out to a buoy, turn left, and continue to another buoy a little less than half a mile south, and then round that buoy and swim back toward the starting area, where they would turn right at the final buoy and head back to the beach from which they started.

Pete and Geraldine were in the back of the pack, but moving steadily. Since the race was parallel to shore, I knew that they could swim in any time they wished. The race organizers and the lifeguards drove the lifeguard truck along the beach toward the south turn buoy to be ready to help if needed.

Pete and Geraldine rounded the buoy successfully!

The leading swimmers were already running through the finish chute, and before long the finish line would be taken down, but Pete and Geraldine were still swimming. A little beyond the turn buoy, I saw them turn in toward shore, a half mile down the beach from the starting line.

Richard, who had already finished the race, and I walked there to cheer them on and hug them as they waded up through the surf into the soft sand.

"Hurray, you made it!" I shouted as I embraced Pete.

He smiled and said, "I was able to help her along."

No one ever mentioned that, of course, it was Geraldine who was helping Pete and not the other way around. No one ever mentioned that they had come to shore in the middle of the race after the finish gate was closed down. She had slowed down her speed and accommodated her pace to swim next to him. What a friend!

She told me later that the lifeguards kept worriedly checking on the two of them, because of their slow progress. When she finally began feeling the cold herself, she told Pete, that because of some big swells coming in the lifeguards on the jet ski were cutting the race short.

Pete looked shoreward, and right on cue, a big set of waves crashed, so he said to Geraldine, "The lifeguards are right! They are smart and we should follow their orders."

On shore, Geraldine thanked Pete for letting her swim with him, and he told her it had been his pleasure to be able to help her out.

When I look back on this day, I realize how many friends helped us out, and in all kinds of ways. Our friends, knowing the daily stress I was dealing with, went out of their way to help me. What would I have done without them? No one wants to face these life-changing situations alone. Let your friends help you!

Pets

Pets can help in so many ways. In our case, our dog Bella helped us. She is a Labrador Retriever with an extraordinarily affectionate personality. Pete had not been a dog person to begin with, but Bella made a big difference for him.

Because of Bella, Pete and I took many more walks in the neighborhood than we might have without her. This gave Pete exercise, but an even more important aspect of having Bella was that the walks gave Pete the opportunity to meet and talk with the neighbors. Pete thoroughly enjoyed starting up conversations with all kinds of people.

And for me, Bella was a godsend. Her loving nature kept me grounded, and her nuzzles and wet kisses buoyed my spirits on a daily basis. I highly recommend having a dog or cat handy when you are caregiving. A short snuggle with a dog or cat is good medicine for the caregiver.

Time Together

I tried to use many "special joys" as a way to keep us close. Now that Pete is gone, I treasure the memories of these moments even more. Caregiving is tough, but it has its highlights and I will cherish the memories we made together after his diagnosis as well as the ones before his diagnosis.

One of the treasures of caregiving memories is that they often center on seemingly small activities. For instance, finding television shows that interested Pete made me feel great. He loved "Downton Abbey" and "The Roosevelts." I taped them, and since twenty minutes of watching was enough for him, I would then show them to him in small portions. He particularly liked the old newsreel clips of FDR with the upturned jaunty cigarette holder, and every time I see such photos, I will think of Pete.

He had been an avid reader. As his LBD progressed, he found lengthy reading difficult, so I would read entire books aloud to him. As with the television shows, we did this in small portions. Sometimes I would read to him in bed, so I could put my arm around him while I read.

As a side note, I found that touching and snuggling were essential – for me and for Pete. There is something about a warm hug and a kiss that can't be duplicated any other way. I lavished affection on Pete, my lovable big guy.

I also found that music was a great healer. I would play CDs of his favorite music, like the Irish Tenors or old favorite tunes, like "Moon River." Sometimes I played the music as a background for our reading, and other times I would just snuggle my head into Pete's chest and we would listen together.

Many studies have shown that music has a powerful therapeutic effect on patients with memory issues. I encouraged him to sing along, and then complimented him, "You can remember the words to all those old songs!"

SELF CARE
Support groups

I can't say enough about support groups. I found a monthly one at UCSD, not too far from home. Before we got to the point where I could not leave Pete alone at home, I attended some sessions. At first I went with questions and a little apprehension about what the group could give to me, and what I could give to them. I found that meeting others who faced similar or worse situations helped me cope with many caregiver issues.

Fortified with Kleenex, we sat in a circle. Tracey, the facilitating social worker, asked each of us to say briefly why we were there, whom we were caring for and what his/her particular challenges were. Each member of the group received practical and emotional support from the facilitator and other caregivers. Most importantly, I quickly realized that I was not alone. I also found it was as beneficial for me to explain my own situation as it was to listen to the situations of others.

The group met monthly, focusing jointly on LBD and Fronto-Temporal Dementia, since the two share some behavioral symptoms. Some attendees, especially those new to the group, were in tears as they spoke about their loved one facing difficult issues. Truly, only others who are also dealing with the daily dilemmas of dementia care for a loved one can fully understand the challenges.

Tracey was well versed in dementia care, and I learned many things. For instance, that Pete's voluntary willing-ness to give up driving was uncommon, but that his sleep disturbances and emotional highs and lows were issues that affected many LBD patients. She had lots of suggestions and solutions for practical as well as mental and emotional issues.

I found that many members of the group faced graver problems than I did. My heart broke for a woman there who at my age was a caregiver for her daughter, a Fronto-Temporal Dementia patient in her fifties.

So many of the questions that had been bouncing around inside of me were asked and answered: What sorts of disposable underwear were the most absorbent? Which kinds could be taken off and on without removing one's shoes and pants? What should I tell my loved one about his disease? When he has delusions or hallucinations, should I correct him and explain that they are not real, or should I play along with what he says? When his paranoia causes him to accuse his caregiver of some wrongdoing (marital infidelity being a common one), how should I deal with those issues?

~ ~ ~

When I left for the support group meetings, I would tell Pete "I'm going to a monthly meeting to learn more about Lewy Body Dementia."

"I want to come with you," he said. He wanted to learn more about his own disease, so was disappointed when I told him the group was for supporters instead of patients. I learned later that there are many opportunities for caregivers and patients to attend groups as a pair. If

I had recognized Pete's condition earlier we both could have benefitted from attending.

By the time I found this information, Pete's was beyond that capability. Nonetheless, going to this support group helped me a lot, and talking about it with Pete afterward was helpful too.

Dementia Wives

I loved the support group I found at UCSD, but I also dearly valued an informal support group we called Dementia Wives. I joined Pat and Gail, all of us with Navy veteran husbands with similar illnesses, and started an occasional lunch gathering. They too provided all the benefits of caring support, and additionally understood what those Navy men were all about!

~5~
LABOR DAY WEEKEND

A ONE-TWO PUNCH
Punch One

One of the things I learned about caregiving is that just as you settle into what looks like a situation you can handle, things can change quickly. I felt as if Pete and I had quite successfully made the transition to taking care of him at home, but LBD is progressive, and at one point a very difficult night and a startling wakeup call changed everything.

On Friday, August 30, Pete had a very bad night. His muscle control had been exhibiting signs of extreme tension, but I had always been able to assuage the tightness through massage and other calming techniques.

"Stretch out your legs and close your eyes," I whispered calmly in his ear, while caressing his arms and legs.

He would listen for a few seconds but soon his body would clench and tighten again. I could almost hear his mind racing as I tried to calm him. His leg muscles were wound up tightly, like a pitcher's arm getting ready to hurl a fastball. I stroked his calf and lowered his leg to the bed, but it would immediately pop up again. The same was true of his head. Even as I repeated soothing words and stroked his forehead, he kept jerking his head up off the pillow. He seemed like a feverish baby not able to let his limbs unwind and rest.

It was late into the night when Pete finally fell sleep on top of the sheets and blankets, and I could finally rest and get a little sleep myself.

I had called Dr. Speckart early on Friday evening. It had been more than six months since I initially talked with him. Both Pete and I had decided not to use drugs to relax his muscles, but luckily I had some on hand, per Dr. Speckart's advice. Now Pete obviously needed some drugs to relieve muscle tension, but that night, they made no difference.

Luckily, Dr. Speckart, a compassionate human being as well as a superb physician, had made himself personally available via cell phone, starting at 5 A.M. any morning. I had avoided calling him so early in the morning before, respecting his privacy and knowing how busy he was. That Saturday, I called him at 5 A.M. telling him that I had never seen Pete like this, truly unable to "let go."

Unfortunately, it was just before the start of a busy Labor Day weekend holiday, so Dr. Speckart advised bringing Pete to the Emergency Room, but wanted to wait till after the holiday weekend, because the emergency rooms would be busy then with casualties from drinking and beach accidents. Also, Dr. Speckart thought Pete's thinking would be sharper if we came to the hospital early in the morning.

I resigned myself to waiting until Tuesday morning, September 3rd. The wait was interminable, giving my already frazzled brain and heart more and more worries.

I was also extremely tired. Pete had not slept through an entire night in weeks now. This, of course, meant that I had not gotten a full night's sleep either. I was worried that I might fall asleep and leave Pete unsupervised. The "long" on this long weekend would indeed be long.

After my call with Dr. Speckart, I went back to bed. Pete was sleeping, exhausted. I looked at his now calm face, and cried. It was just a small cry. In reality, I was too exhausted for a full out sob, and because of my role as his caregiver, going down that road was something I avoided. While I am a huge advocate of self-care for caregivers, there are points where you just need to focus and get through. That weekend was one of those points.

Punch Two

I started Saturday morning telling myself, "You can do this!"

Punch two came late that morning...

I still feel blessed that I decided to poke my head in to check on Pete – just in time. He was in the bathroom, in front of the sink.

"Good morning," I chirped, pretending to be carefree. I'm going to make you pancakes for breakfast today. Your favorite!"

He was looking down, concentrating on his task at hand, and he did not answer my greeting.

I looked down to see what he was focused on and saw that he was putting his toothpaste on his razor. His razor!

After the very rough Friday night, any resistance I had to taking Pete into the hospital as soon as possible was released when I realized what he was doing. Not wanting him to know how dangerous that was, I quietly cleaned it off and reminded him what razors and toothbrushes were for, and what they needed—shaving lotion and toothpaste—to do their jobs.

Right underneath my calm was a panic. I realized that I could not monitor him every minute of the day and night. I could not, on my own, keep him safe. The time had come. Friday night and Saturday morning showed me that the days of my managing his needs by myself at home had come to an end. It became clear that this was a turning point.

A BIG DECISION

The events of Friday night and Saturday morning had really made the decision, but I still had to let my mind catch up. I also needed to talk things over with Katherine and Susan, Pete's daughters. I had the rest of the holiday weekend for both of these tasks.

With Katherine and Susan's help and input, we worked out the next steps together. We all knew that after I took him into the emergency room, he would go to a care center. They both made arrangements to fly in over the following week to help me with the transition.

Meanwhile, my heart kept screaming at me when I thought about Pete in a memory care facility. My Pete, needing to be cared for in a facility? How could I do this to him? Yet I saw no way that I could take care of him at home, even with full-time help, which wasn't even an option for us.

This decision to move Pete to a memory care facility was a big one, filled with lots of emotion but weighed down with common sense. I thought back on what I had learned through my many years of swim races. I had learned how to both lose and win gracefully. This felt like both a loss and a win. The thought of not having him at home was excruciating, but the peace of mind from knowing that he would be safe and cared for felt like relief.

~6~
TUESDAY MORNING: THE HOSPITAL

THE EMERGENCY ROOM

The first step in Pete's transition to a care facility was the emergency room. Unfortunately, even if you have doctors following your case, the emergency room is often the easiest and quickest way to get someone admitted to the hospital. This is a strange quirk of the medical system. So as instructed by our doctor, I would take Pete to the emergency room on Tuesday, the day after Labor Day.

Tuesday couldn't come soon enough. I woke before 6 A.M. and got Pete ready. I tried not to think about how big this day was going to be. Several times I was tempted to just sit down and cry, but I kept up a cheerful attitude for Pete. I got up, got dressed quickly, made a simple breakfast for Pete. It hit me that this might be the last breakfast I made for Pete in this kitchen. I was so nervous that I could hardly eat.

At breakfast I finally told Pete that we were going to the emergency room and that he might stay in the hospital. I don't know if he understood or not, but he smiled and said "That's a good plan." While I will never know if he meant what he said, it did make me feel better.

~ ~ ~

The emergency room doctor started by asking Pete, "Who is the President of the U.S.? What day is it today?" Pete's unknowing responses proved that the LBD was truly taking a toll.

A staff member from the hospital's behavioral unit was called in. She asked him if he would be willing to be admitted as a patient and he agreed. Again, I am not sure if he understood what he was agreeing to or not, but he had to be admitted.

She then took me aside, and in a quiet voice told me, "We are overcrowded in the behavioral ward here, so we might have to send him to another hospital, like the Naval Hospital in San Diego."

This was upsetting. I knew that for Dr. Speckart to see him, he should be at this hospital, and I found myself insisting that they keep him there. An important part of caregiving is standing up for your loved ones in such situations. This can be particularly challenging in hospital and care situations, but it is crucial.

As it happened, there was one available bed, but it was in the acute care area of the behavioral ward. This meant that his shoelaces and belt would be taken away from him. In this ward, patients could not have anything on them that could be potentially dangerous.

This was not the way I envisioned him entering a care facility. To start Pete off in such a harsh situation frightened me, but at this point, there was no better choice.

This then brought me to the scene I described at the beginning of this book. The scene that still haunts me to this day. I was devastated and shocked at how quickly I lost control once we entered the hospital. The staff was great, and I believe they were looking out for our best choices, but it was still overwhelming. This was the lowest point for me. For Pete, scared and locked up. For me, helpless in caring for Pete.

THE ACUTE CARE WARD

The psychiatric staff in the Acute Care Ward wanted to keep him in the hospital until his condition stabilized, which turned out to be five or six days. I knew he was in good hands, but this behavioral ward was not where he belonged. It was scary and intense.

Visiting hours were only between 7 and 8 pm. We had to go through two locked entrances to get to where he was. There were always patients in the hallways, just pacing up and down, some sullen, some jabbering away, others shouting. Its plain walls and locked doors made it feel like an institution from an old horror movie.

To this day I am upset that he had to stay there at all. I tried to get him moved to another ward, but to no avail. I went from being a caregiver at home, carrying the full burden, but also having the control over how Pete was cared for, to being helpless.

When his daughter Susan arrived the day after he was admitted, we both agonized over this situation, but we also kept reassuring ourselves that even though this acute behavioral ward was forbidding, it was only a way station. In fact, it doubled my resolve to find him a care facility that could truly be a new home for him.

While all of this was happening, I have to note that the night Pete was admitted to the hospital was the first night in a long time that I had a full and uninterrupted night of sleep. While I was heartbroken to sleep alone, there was some relief to being able to sleep a full night without immediate worries about his safety. This is, of course, not to say that there wasn't some tossing and turning about all the other things that were going on.

Surprisingly, through all of this, Pete remained peaceful about his situation. Perhaps his sense of place or belonging was already compromised. In any event, I was intensely proud of him.

~7~
PETE'S NEW HOME

CHOOSING A CARE FACILITY

While I hated that Pete was in the Acute Care Ward, it gave me the chance to choose a care facility and make all the arrangements. Luckily I had already done some research, but now it was real.

Choosing a care facility is not easy. There are so many issues to balance and it is unlikely that you will find the perfect place for the perfect amount of money.

I must admit, it is also easy to put a lot of pressure on the "perfect" part. For me, quite honestly, I realize now that a mixture of my love for Pete, and some guilt about moving him out of our home and into a care center, made me try for perfect. Eventually, you find someplace that can become a home for your loved one, and it does not have to be absolutely perfect.

That said, we did find a great place where Pete was very well taken care of, and the "angels" on that staff will have my gratitude forever.

I believe it is also difficult to choose the care facility because yet again you are making an important decision for your loved one, and making it without his or her input. I was lucky that Pete and I had visited some retirement and care centers before we even got the diagnosis, and to make things easier for me, I remembered that Pete had had positive things to say about our visit to the Coronado Retirement Village.

This doesn't mean that my choice was completely easy. I also gathered all the recommendations I could from friends. My Dementia Wives were particularly helpful. And true to my nature, I visited each care center with a list of questions and a keen eye for what I liked and didn't like.

When I entered the Coronado Retirement Village, I took note of how clean, modern, and appealing the center was. I also noticed the enclosed rear garden, showcasing a view of San Diego Bay, providing a place where guests and residents could gather. Although he couldn't go to the outside gardens on his own, I was free to take him there. I liked that I could envision myself sitting in that garden with him.

THE LOCKED-UP FACTOR

One of the biggest benefit of having Pete in a care facility was that he would be safe and monitored 24/7. Yet the locked-up factor of the memory care unit was a sticking point in my mind. Pete would not have free access to all the grounds; he would not be allowed to walk to the village; he would not even be allowed downstairs without another adult. I wasn't sure how Pete would react to this, but I did know that he needed supervision and could not be left on his own.

I felt better when I was told that a third of the residents who were in the memory care unit, behind those locked doors and on the second floor, didn't even realize they were locked up. Plus, there were multiple opportunities for residents in the memory care unit to be brought downstairs, and to go outdoors for activities, including exercise classes, word games, and musical presentations. More active residents could also be taken downstairs for meals in the big dining room, rather than eating upstairs with residents who were less able to feed themselves and less able to communicate. There were even planned "field trips," that I could tag along on.

Additionally, I could take Pete home or on our own outings as often and long as I chose. His friends could take Pete out for activities or meals too.

So I added all of this together with the fact that they had an available room, and the facility was only seven minutes from our home. With great relief, I said "yes" to Pete having a new home.

~~~

I do want to make a note here: financially, Pete and I were very lucky. Pete's own careful planning had made this move possible, and I was overwhelmingly grateful. His long-term health care policy paid for much of his care at the center and there was little financial burden until the last few months of his life, when his disease worsened and his care needs escalated. I mention this because this is not true for everyone and I want to recognize that financial challenges at times like these make everything more difficult. My heart goes out to caregivers who have to add financial worries to the mix.

OUT OF THE HOSPITAL, INTO THE CARE CENTER

While he was in the Acute Care Ward, I could only visit Pete for one hour a day. As I mentioned, this gave me the time to finalize plans for a care center for Pete, but it also gave me time to worry myself with questions: "If he is not living with me at home, will he feel deserted when he wakes up during the night? Will he miss me? How will we move him there? How will we get his favorite rocking chair there? What about his clothing? What about his belongings? Am I ready to handle all the physical and emotional issues that will certainly come up?"

From the perspective of now looking back, I would advise caregivers not to spend so much time worrying about such details. Some things just take care of themselves, and as for the others, you can face them if and when they show up. One thing I discovered was that many of the professionals, at the hospital and the care center, have the experience to guide you through or take care of things for you. Let them!

For instance, while Pete was in the behavioral ward, I contacted the director of the retirement facility we had selected. The director then went to visit Pete in the behavioral ward and talked with him about moving to their facility. This kindness softened the blow of this big move for Pete, and for me. She also arranged for him to be taken to the care center by ambulance.

~ ~ ~

While we waited for Pete to be let out of the Acute Care Ward, we were given access to his room at the care center. Katherine and Susan flew in and joined me in making the room welcoming, comfortable, and homelike. We hung framed artwork by his grandchildren on the walls. We displayed old framed newspaper articles, including one featuring a leaping Pete catching a football at a Harvard-Yale game. We populated the bookshelf and the desk with photographs of laughing happy children and grandchildren. We brought his favorite cookies and his most loved comfortable clothes, especially t-shirts reminding him of past physical conquests. With the help of a borrowed truck, we were able to move everything he needed to the facility, even his favorite rocking chair, which I had spent time worrying about.

In many ways, preparing his room was a high point. Together, his daughters and I felt like we were doing something for him, something that would make him happy despite the circumstances.

~8~
SETTLING IN

THE MEMORY CARE UNIT

The good news was that because of Pete's resilient attitude and social nature, his stay in the retirement facility began smoothly. Even though he had mental relapses, his basic personality remained intact.

I worried about how the staff and other residents would react to him? I so wanted them to see what a superb person he was. Therefore, I became very proactive in creating relationships with the staff and other residents. These relationships are worth their weight in gold, and will benefit you and your loved ones, and make things better for the staff and other residents too. Additionally, getting to know the other visiting families is beneficial.

Seeing the diminished state in which many residents lived—not being able to talk or walk, for instance—cut me to the bone. It worried me that Pete would slide into such a static state. I resolved to spend as much time as possible with him, so that I could keep his brain active. During the first days of decorating his room I made plans in my head to keep bringing him news and interesting articles. I would take him outside on walks. I would show him pictures of his family. We would discuss memories from our past.

I would also keep our love strong. In fact, since the staff took care of his daily needs such as bathing, eating, and exercising, I no longer had to personally worry about his entire well-being, and I could more fully tend to his emotional needs.

I also planned to bring him home for many visits, although I must admit, it felt strange to think in terms of bringing my husband "home for a visit."

I soon realized that this decision was the right one. Having him in the care center would keep him safe, and I must admit, I felt the relief of not having the entire burden of his care and safety resting on me. So this felt right, and yet, I missed hugging him as I fell asleep, and I missed turning to him as I woke up. I missed the smell of him in bed. I missed the weight of his body next to mine.

The Gym

Timing was in our favor. They were in the process of outfitting a mini gym for the residents, just as we arrived at the care center. This was perfect for Pete.

While I had talked to Pete about his diagnosis being more serious than the original Mild Cognitive Impairment, he told me that "If I just work harder and exercise more, I can get better." So despite telling him he had LBD, which is incurable, I encouraged him to "work harder." After all, hope is a wonderful thing, and if nothing else, makes us feel better.

Since the gym was located outside the locked area, someone needed to take Pete there. We met the on-site physical therapist, John, and he immediately struck up a friendship with Pete, and went out of his way to make sure Pete got to visit the gym. While helping Pete work out, John obviously enjoyed chatting with Pete about last weekend's football or baseball game. Since Pete loved to chat with friends and neighbors about what the world out there was up to, I was grateful that John, this energetic and likable young man, was genuinely interested in Pete. He asked Pete all kinds of questions about his Navy and athletic career. John was truly a significant factor in making Pete's transition to assisted living more palatable.

MY NEW ROLE

Pete's move into a care center transformed both Pete's life and mine. Between the long Labor Day Weekend of worry and the time Pete had to spend in the Acute Care Ward, it was a rough nine days. And now, a new stage in our LBD journey.

Another Rabbit Hole

The original recognition of Pete's LBD was the first "rabbit hole." As Pete moved into the care facility, it felt like we were falling down another rabbit hole, into the unknowable and the illogical. A door was definitely closing on our previous life. There was little clarity about what would happen next.

Interestingly enough, it is often the caregivers who feels like their own responsibilities and feelings are being transformed, even more than those of their loved ones. Especially in cases of dementia, our loved ones are often a bit oblivious to the changes. Pete seemed accepting of his new "home," whereas I was filled with all those questions and worries. Indeed, these rabbit holes may just be more difficult for the caregivers to navigate.

Luckily, I had been tending to the reservoir of love that I mentioned at the beginning. Having that to draw from helped me deal with the new challenges, and made me a better caregiver. I was able to stay heart-centered in my care for Pete. I was determined to stay in love with

Pete, and to infuse everything I did for and with him with love.

Doing this would again mean activating all the lessons I had learned through long distance swimming. I would pace myself. I would keep myself nourished. I would welcome support. I would be prepared for the unknown. I would persevere. I would keep up a steady rhythm. I would enjoy the sights along the way, and embrace each small and large joy, even within the challenges.

I told myself, "You can do this."

Guilt

At first, visiting my husband at a "facility" felt artificial compared to our previous life together. This made me feel quite guilty at times. Although I knew in my heart of hearts that it was the right place for him, I still felt guilty about not taking care of him in our home. It did not matter that I knew this was the most loving thing I could do for him – I still felt guilty, and I imagine that there will be a little guilt about this inside of me for the rest of my life. I accept it.

~9~

A NEW NORMAL

MY VISITS TO THE CARE CENTER

I did two things to make my visits better for me and for Pete. I brought our dog Bella with me as often as possible. When Bella went with me to visit Pete, everyone was happy.

The second thing I did was to truly open up to enjoying the care center activities myself. We were participating for Pete's sake, but I found myself looking forward to the activities too.

Bella Love

She was always excited to see Pete and would jump up onto his bed and smother him with wet kisses. Pete felt the love! Bella also gave us a great way to interact with the other patients. Even those who were less communicative would smile and want to pet her.

Also, just as he used to use Bella as an excuse to start conversation with our neighbors, Pete now used Bella as a conversation starter with other patients, staff, and visitors. Pete was already popular at the center, but Bella raised his "status" even higher.

Many facilities have program where they bring dogs in, and I applaud that. I would also say that bringing a pet your loved one already knows is even better. But either way, dogs are love, and I truly believe that Bella helped both Pete and me through our "long distance swim" with LBD.

Care Center Activities

I came to cherish the special morning activities at the center. For instance, on Wednesdays an old-fashioned piano player and crooner would play and sing in the living room downstairs. For LBD patients, hearing old tunes from their pasts, and remembering the song lyrics, are great activities. I would set my chair right next to Pete's so I could hold his hand while we listened. Pete loved the fact that he was the one often asked for song suggestions, and the others in the room loved Pete's wonderful baritone voice.

Over time, these events and others made me realize that while things had changed, we had found a new way to be together, and while it was different from what we had, it was still filled with love, and we could still enjoy ourselves fully.

OUT AND ABOUT

Home Visits

I brought Pete home as often as possible. At first I worried that he wouldn't want to return to the care facility. That turned out not to be an issue After watching a few segments of a television show, or catching a sporting event on television, he would take a brief nap, then tell me, "I'm ready to go back now." At first I felt a bit disappointed by his desire to go back, but I realized that it was where he was comfortable now. The good news was that it had become "home" for him.

"Field Trips"

Especially at the beginning of his stay at the care center, we had lots of outings. We often met friends for lunch, and this made Pete, a natural storyteller who loved an audience, very happy. Planning outings that complement your loved one's assets and interests is "good medicine" for LBD patients.

Interest-wise, Pete was a big sports fans, so when the care center offered a trip to see a San Diego Padres baseball game, I jumped at the chance to sign us up to go. Because music seemed to make Pete feel better, I sought out local concerts. Because Pete had served in Vietnam, I took him to hear a presentation from an admiral who had been held captive in Hanoi during the Vietnam War.

While I was always looking for activities that Pete and I would enjoy, I was also being a "strategic" caregiver. I looked for activities that would ignite Pete's memories in positive ways.

Swimming

I continued to take Pete to early morning swim workouts three times a week. The care center staff must have thought me nuts to drive up at 5 am, but they gallantly unlocked the front door, knowing that Pete would be ready to go.

We would get to the UCSD pool before 5:45, so Pete could fulfill his perennial desire to be the first person there, and the first person to help take the tarps off the pool before the workout. As a member of a SEAL team, the values of punctuality and of being helpful to others were instilled in him. Getting him to the pool fifteen minutes before the start of the practice allowed Pete to feel in synch with his values. This was as much a part of his care as anything else I could have done for him.

Going to this swim workout had always been important for Pete, and we continued to go as far into his illness as possible.

Hooyah!

Irish Flynn, one of Pete's Navy friends, took Pete to a swim workout two days a week, on Wednesdays and Fridays. Not only did this give Pete some "guy time," but it was also special because they swam at the Naval Amphibious Base, where they could watch the SEAL team trainees and talk with them, giving them the traditional "hooyah" support cheer. Irish, not being a long-time swimmer himself, even called Pete "Coach Pete," a moniker that always brought a smile to Pete's face.

This was not only a gift to Pete, but also to me. This gave me two free mornings to catch up on other things. Irish was my "wing man" on those early morning swim practices.

~10~
TAKING CARE OF PETE

UNDERSTANDING
HIS LEWY BODY DEMENTIA

Lewy Body Dementia is not as well known as Alzheimer's, but is the second most common progressive dementia. As mentioned earlier, LBD also has an overlap with Parkinson's, bringing symptoms such as speech and motor function difficulties. There are still many open questions about LBD, and it can only be definitively diagnosed at autopsy. The disease is progressive and the adding up of symptoms pushed relentlessly forward on Pete.

Mental Functioning

Mentally, Pete, who had been known as a leader both in the Navy community and as a Juvenile Court judge, struggled with his "executive functions." It was more and more difficult for him to make a plan and execute it. I soon developed a habit of repeating myself many times. Repetition can be reassuring for someone with LBD.

One important tool that helped Pete was a white board. I wrote out a daily schedule for him. This proved to be both very helpful and reassuring to Pete. Although, there was sometimes one hitch: Pete would erase the board. If he did erase the board, he would keep calling me to find out what he was supposed to do next.

Eventually, I had to turn off the ringer on my phone at night, because Pete would call me numerous times to check on his schedule. I gave the care center my cell phone number so they could call me in the case of an emergency.

Worries

Throughout our marriage, his worries were my worries and vice versa. Now his worries were my worries, but in a very different way.

Worries often crop up in areas where the LBD patient has worried before. Since personal responsibility and punctuality were always central for Pete, it was no surprise that it was often in those areas that his worries occurred. I found that changing the subject was often a simple and useful strategy to deflect his worries. Or I would talk about or read something that triggered a positive emotional memory. These were good agitation deflectors.

Emotional Shifts and Delusions

One of the most difficult issues for me was his emotional shifts and delusions. Earlier I mentioned his most common delusion about some boyfriend he thought I had. One minute he would be accusing me of meeting or talking with this boyfriend, and the next minute he would be himself again, apologizing to me. I must admit that even when I knew he would be quickly shifting back to reality, it was difficult to let myself be accused of infidelity. Similar stories from others at the support group helped a lot.

Another delusion that he would have was that I was another Betsy, not Betsy his wife. I remember the first time I heard him telling my daughter Amy that there were two Betsys. Eventually he told both of his daughters and all of his stepchildren about this other Betsy. Apparently, one Betsy was his wife. The other was some sort of bad person. According to him, this other Betsy would often keep talking to him while he was watching a movie. "I'm in a movie theater and there is this woman who won't be quiet so I can watch the movie!"

As with the infidelity delusion, this idea of two Betsys had started before he went to live at the care center, but did continue throughout his illness. He once told a neighbor, "This is not my wife!" "I'm married to the other Betsy!" I ended up asking the neighbor to come into our house so she could point out, in our wedding photos and in the framed wedding certificate on the wall in the living room, that I was indeed his wife. Eventually, I learned to "go with the flow," and not even try to convince Pete that there were not two Betsys… or a boyfriend.

Some of the delusions were not so bad. One of Pete's imaginary court cases got him to the Supreme Court. In the memory care unit, he would pepper his talk with typical court words, like "Ladies and gentlemen, the court will now come to order." Some residents humored him, and asked him to legislate questions or pound an imaginary gavel on a table.

Correcting an LBD sufferer with facts is often less successful than playing along. For instance, he would telephone me and tell me "I am on a train and I don't know where I am supposed to get off," or "I'm on a ship and no one will tell me where we are going." At first I tried rationality and told him "Well, since you are calling me from your room, I think it is likely that you are not on a ship." Eventually I just told him he was traveling by ship to Hawaii.

Admittedly, at times I found it difficult not to try to understand a particular delusion. For instance, why would Pete imagine or think up this idea of two Betsys? And it is true that I felt a bit bruised by his accusations of infidelity, even though I knew they were only imagined.

Drowsiness and Fainting

LBD is also difficult for the caregiver because there are physical symptoms. Increasingly, Pete would experience daytime drowsiness and fainting. This meant that he could even fall asleep while sitting or walking.

Since Pete was six-foot-five, this meant that I had to be even more vigilant as a caregiver. When he got drowsy or fainted, his weight could easily overwhelm my physical ability to hold and guide him.

Eventually it became clear that outings needed to be short and not include too many stops. On one occasion, when Irish had taken him out for breakfast after swimming, Pete fell so soundly asleep at the restaurant table that Irish had to enlist a strong young restaurant employee to carry him to the car. At one point, taking Pete to swimming and breakfast became just a trip to the pool. I am thankful that Pete did not fall asleep while swimming!

Muscle Weakness and Rigidity

LBD takes its toll in obvious physical ways. You will remember that one of the wake-up calls that led to moving

Pete into a care center appeared when I could no longer control the muscle spasms and rigidity that would take over his legs and arms. At the care center, Pete could be on medicine that would help calm his muscles. This could add to his drowsiness, but at the care center there were health aides to help him move around.

Drug Side Effects

Not surprisingly, Pete's medical care included medications, including the muscle relaxers just mentioned. As a caregiver, it is good to be informed about medications. I would research the drugs online and talk with other caregivers and social workers at the LBD support groups. From my research, I could then ask the doctors educated questions about the drugs and their side effects.

Knowing side effects is key. I was surprised to find out that some drugs are contraindicated for LBD and can even hasten death. We used anti-psychotic drugs to combat Pete's anxiety and agitation, but they also lowered his blood pressure. At a point, the "cushion" they gave Pete was worth the dangerous side effects.

The drugs also added to Pete's risk of falling from either drowsiness or fainting. The timing and size of doses can be crucial, with smaller doses during the daytime and larger doses at night.

TALKING TO PETE ABOUT LBD

We all wondered how much Pete understood about his own situation. I tried to tell him about LBD. I wanted him to know that he was living where he was because he needed supervision and medication. With dementia conditions, you can never be sure what your loved one truly understands. At some points, I felt as if he understood what I was telling him, but then shortly afterward, he would say something that seemed to indicate he didn't understand his situation at all.

I think he knew it was a serious disease—and he must have had some inkling that it was progressive and eventually lethal—but he chose to talk about it as if it were a challenge that he was attempting to overcome. He thought that way about the medications too. "If I could just take more of this medicine I would be much better!" he would say. I tried to gently explain to him that more medicine would not make him better, but I admired his tenacity.

I did tell Pete that at the microscopic level, there are actually Lewy Bodies. Specifically, they are protein deposits. Pete sometimes referred to these Lewy Bodies as brain gremlins named "Louie," while tapping his head and blaming "Louie" for what was happening. His quirky sense of humor stayed with him!

CARING WITH LOVE

When Pete accused me of having a boyfriend or being the other Betsy, I responded with hugs and assurances that he was the only man for me and that I was the luckiest woman in the world to be married to him. When he erased the day's schedule on his white board, I rewrote it. When he couldn't think something through, I reminded myself that this was a mission of love

The fact that he had been slowed down by this disease actually heightened my love and compassion for him. After all, he had not asked for this to happen to him. In fact, he had always taken superb care of himself, so this seemed very unfair. But I could not spend a lot of time on the unfairness.

I also realized that just as he was being transformed by LBD, so too was I. In fact, I was becoming a stronger and even more loving wife, and taking care of Pete was something I did with great love.

~11~
MY PETE

While the symptoms of LBD are the same for everyone, each person will react differently to the disease, and each will have specific ways in which LBD manifests itself. As caregivers, I think that we are always looking for the places where our loved one's unique personality breaks through the fog of the disease.

I loved it when I saw "my Pete," the Pete I met and married, shine through his illness. I also did everything I could to help that Pete come through. One of the most important things caregivers can do is to praise and encourage their loved ones in a positive and proactive way.

HELPING OTHERS

I was touched to hear that Pete, when he heard some commotion outside his room, went to the door and asked "May I be of assistance, ma'am?" It was vintage Pete— always wanting to help others. His many years as a juvenile court judge finely attuned him to the psychological and physical needs of others. I knew it was empowering for him to continue his altruistic endeavors, so I encouraged him, telling him how much he was helping others. He could then keep feeling like the old Pete, and I could keep appreciating him for that.

NO WHINING

Even given all that attention, Pete must have been lonely inside. His face would light up when I arrived, but he never complained. That of course was the key to the SEAL team "No whining" philosophy. I remembered the SEAL shirt he had once given me emblazoned with the SEAL team motto" "The only easy day was yesterday." Now he was living that motto.

HIS SENSE OF HUMOR

Throughout his illness Pete kept his sense of humor— both about the illness itself and raconteur status he had always been known for. I imagine that at times, this was a true inner struggle for Pete. I applaud him for bringing out "the real Pete" so often. I also did everything I could to encourage that funny, witty, storyteller husband I knew and loved.

"Judge, did you swim this morning?" a retirement center staff member asked Pete one day. His quick answer: "Does a bear sleep in the woods?" This was pure Pete!

Sometimes—not always--he realized that he had delusions, and he might begin a sentence with "This may be one of my delusions, but...."

Once, he said to me with a smile, "Now about these delusions. We could have some fun with that. If I eat an illusionary hamburger, will I gain illusionary weight?" This was one of my all-time favorite Pete remarks. I treasured those occasional flashes of brilliance. To this day, everyone laughs when I tell this story.

I share this about my husband knowing that the situation will not be the same for everyone – but I will say, that as caregivers, while LBD may be a horrendously debilitating "foe," we can take seemingly small steps in the way we take care of our loved ones and these small steps will make all the difference in the world. Throughout our LBD journey, I was there to laugh at his jokes and enjoy his wit. I truly believe I was giving him great medicine with every laugh and smile.

PETE'S LOVE OF WORDS

Since I wasn't sleeping as well as I would like, I thought about going to the 7:30 a.m. swim workout instead of the 6 a.m. This reminded me that years earlier I had told Pete that when we both retired we could go to the 7:30 workout.

"Going at 7:30," he said, "would be slothful!"

When Irish Flynn started taking him to swim on Wednesdays and Fridays, I was free to go to my own UCSD workouts at 7:30 am on those days. When I told Pete that I was thinking about going to the 7:30 swim workout, a twinkle came to his eye and he said, "A life of sloth!" His love of words and his sense of humor were definitely linked.

After telling my swim friends this story, they said "Hello, Mrs. Sloth," when I showed up at the 7:30 a.m. workouts.

~~~

As I look back I also realize that Pete's sustaining wit gave me great stories to tell the many people that cared about him, and this buoyed me as a caregiver. For instance, Ellen, a swim friend, sent good wishes to Pete and added, "if he remembers me."

I passed this message on to Pete, and he said with a smile "Of COURSE I remember her! I am indignant that she thinks I might not remember her. And please tell her that I used that big word "indignant.""

Pete's remark made me look forward to seeing her again so we could laugh together about Pete's response.

PETE'S POPULARITY

This may sound as if I am bragging, but I consider it a fact: Even at 76 years old, Pete was a ruggedly handsome and kind gentleman, and since most of the Memory Care Unit residents were women, he quickly became a popular attraction.

Admittedly, Pete's popularity delighted me a bit. In fact, I felt a wave a disappointment among the female residents when I showed up to visit Pete. Meanwhile, Pete seemed to take it all in stride. After all, before he met me, a local newspaper had written him up as "the most watchable man" in town.

It must have been flattering to him on one level to get all this attention at the care center, but on another level it was a bother for him. The female residents vied for who got to sit next to him in the dining room and came by his room to see him. Some would open his closet and start trying on his shirts, his hats, and even his underwear.

I soon realized that we had entered a whole new world. I now laugh at how like high school it was. There were plenty of small dramas. For instance, there was one woman who, from the back, Pete mistakenly thought was me. When he reached out and touched her arm, her family raised concern about Pete being a "predator." All of this was sorted out, but Pete was embarrassed by it. Then the situation got more complicated because the same woman kept coming by to sit on Pete's bed. Finally, he told her, "Look, I've only known you for two weeks but I've been married to Betsy for almost twenty years!"

This was an aspect of having Pete in assisted living that I did not foresee. I found that as long as I could keep a sense of humor about all of it, it was actually a nice distraction from the more pressing and serious matters of Pete's progressing LBD.

PETE'S FAMILY VALUES

Our children and grandchildren were an important part of Pete's care. Taking care of them was so important to Pete, and as his LBD progressed, he made a graceful transition to letting them look out for him. I installed a phone in his room and pasted up a phone list. Pete did not hesitate to reach out and connect with all of our children.

MOMENTS OF CLARITY

I also want to highlight the moments of clarity that LBD patients can experience. This is one of the perplexing issues of being a caregiver for a person with dementia. To survive you accept a certain vision of how LBD has changed your loved one. Then, quite suddenly, there is a clearing and if someone met him or her at that point, they would not suspect any form of dementia being present.

Once when we were sitting in the waiting room before seeing Dr. Speckart, the conductor of the San Diego Symphony walked in for his flu shot. Pete beamed and said clearly, "Hello, Maestro!"

The maestro beamed too. He sat down near us, and he and Pete carried on a dynamic conversation about the orchestra's upcoming trip to China and about the selections they would be playing at the next concert. Pete was in his element. I am sure that the Maestro walked away thinking that Pete was also there for a mere flu shot.

A SPECIAL EVENT

As a caregiver it is very easy to get bogged down into the basics of caregiving. I have to tell you, now that I am on the other side of things, I so cherish the special moments, big and small, not only from our pre-LBD life, but also our special moments together through his struggles with LBD. As a caregiver, give space to allow for those special moments to happen.

For me, an event I will cherish to the end of my days was our marriage recommitment ceremony. The greatest part of this is that it was Pete's idea. Neither of us ever gave in to the vision of our love being over because of either his illness or his need to be in a memory care facility.

It was a small ceremony, with a few close friends, including Bill Pate, the best man at our wedding twenty years ago, and my sister Judy, who had been matron of honor. Under a sparkling California sky we looked out at the blue bay stretching toward San Diego. Navy ships and smaller boats dotted the harbor and palm trees swayed in the wind. I read "vows" for both of us. I declared that not only did we still love each other, but we loved each other more and more every day.

I looked at Pete – his hair tousled by the wind, his eyes teary with emotion, and his whole being lit up by his smile. I understood that together we would go the distance, however long and however choppy the waves got. I also felt proud of how we were dealing with everything that LBD had thrown at us so far – by answering with love.

I put my arm around Pete and he put his arm around me, and we walked to a nearby gazebo for apple juice and cookies.

~~~

When caregiving an LBD patient, there are always some voices in your head focusing on the descent. Yet to this day, that day was and is a buoy to me. When I feel challenged, I go back to that moment on that sandy bay, and feel such an abundance of love that I feel renewed. This is the power of love, and the power of caregiving with love.

It was a bit sad that after the recommitment ceremony that I had to drive him back to the care facility, and leave him there alone on his narrow bed while I went back to our home alone. But as I went to sleep that night, I relived the day and could still remember the warmth of his comforting body as we sat in the gazebo with our good friends, eating our cookies and drinking our juice.

~12~
THE LAST RACE

A BIG SWIM FOR PETE

Pete and I had been in so many swim races together. We met swimming and we loved to swim together, whether for fun or competition. Swimming was a huge part of our life.

So when Pete wanted to swim an annual Cove-Pier-Cove swim, I understood. Part of me also understood that this would be his last swim.

Our swim coach sponsors this event to give his pool swimmers a chance to swim in the warm summer ocean. One doesn't need to swim the entire mile and a half to the pier and then another mile and a half back, but can do whatever feels right for that person and that day. Pete wanted to swim to the quarter-mile buoy and back.

At first I was overwhelmed with all the reasons why this COULDN'T happen, but then I began musing about how we COULD make it happen. There was a lot to figure out—the steps down to the beach, Pete's slower swimming speed, and his general confusion.

Six good friends volunteered to swim with us and to help him in any way needed, even getting him showered and dressed in the locker room afterward. Up until the day of the swim I worried that this was a lot to ask of friends and maybe I should just tell Pete no. Luckily, one of the lessons learned from caregiving is to let people help me—and so I did.

Seven of us swam right alongside him, stroke for stroke. Everyone was keeping an eye on Pete, but also enjoying the orange garibaldi fish and silver mackerel swimming beneath us. And of course, he was included in the de-rigueur breakfast afterward. The whole event was a real shot in the arm for him!

I am not saying this as a medical professional and completely acknowledge that it is only anecdotal, but I truly believe that Pete's experience of LBD was easier because of events like this. He was surrounded, literally, by people who cared about him, he was challenging himself physically, and he was participating in an event that made him feel like himself again. Just imagine how medicinal this is to an LBD patient.

Unfortunately, as you know, it was his last swim event.

A GRADUAL
BUT VERY REAL DECLINE
Physical Weakness

On the flip side of events like Pete's "Big Swim," I felt helpless as I watched Pete's decline. Physically, Pete was experiencing more dizziness and more episodes of fainting. Falling became a persistent worry. I knew that he could seriously injure himself with a fall. His always-low blood pressure balanced against his anti-psychotic drugs made this a tricky thing to get right.

His motor skills began to tangle up. We added a walker, calling it his "exercise machine." Fatigue weakened him. He welcomed more naps.

There were a growing number of days when I would feel disappointed and frustrated while watching him try to participate in exercises and games at the care center. He was unable to complete the simplest tasks, like putting his ten fingers together and connecting them one by one.

I would try to give him extra instruction, "See, this right hand index finger pairs up with the left hand index finger." Helping him calmed my anxieties, but I am not sure how it felt to Pete. It was just so heartbreaking to see even his basic skills disappearing. He was regressing faster and faster. A thought that he would soon be unable to do anything at all pressed in on me. I did my best to hide that thought and persevere. "Just do what you can," I would reassure him.

Life felt more and more fleeting and tenuous. It was time to deal fully with the reality of his shrinking physical presence.

Cognitive Decline

Pete's troubles with processing and understanding were growing deeper. His characteristic wit and sharpness began to soften. In the situations where I felt as if he understood what was going on, his ability to communicate his thoughts was diminishing. For instance, I brought in and read an article to Pete about a World War II plane. Pete fascination with WWII was rooted in the fact that his father was a pilot during the war. In fact, the plane in the article was the exact kind of plane that his father flew. I knew that Pete connected to this article, but I only knew this because of the tears in his eyes.

Friends and Family

Pete still welcomed letters, notes, and phone calls, as well as visits.

He loved hearing the voices of his daughters. In the late stages of his LBD, when he couldn't really talk, I took the phone out of his room, but I would still hold a cell phone up to his ear so he could hear them.

In some ways, I became a go-between with family and friends who wanted to talk to Pete. I would tell them about his frame of mind or clue them in to other issues before they talked with him. After the calls, my favorite "job" was to deliver hugs to Pete from the people who called. The "hug request" became a favorite sign-off for our grandchildren in particular.

Even when he wanted to talk on the phone and have visitors, I soon realized that I had to be the gatekeeper. He tired easily and I had to keep others from extending the conversations too long. I also came to realize that the anticipation of a phone call or visit was as good as the actual call or visit itself, and less tiring to Pete.

One note that I know other LBD caregivers will understand is that it was a surprise to many that Pete would remember their names. This is one area in which LBD differs from Alzheimer's. His command of names and personal recognition generally continued to be excellent.

CAREGIVING ALL THE WAY

Since Pete's attention span was narrowing, and because he was getting better adjusted to life at the care center, I gradually weaned myself away from spending too much time there. Lengthy visits tended to overload him, so shorter stays seemed a better way to show my love for him. Quality of time, not quantity, was the key.

One activity that Pete continued to love was my reading to him. The closeness of sitting or reclining next to him allowed us some warm touching as well. Sometimes we did this in his room, and sometimes we would sit outside, in the garden or by the front door.

Caregiver Self-Care

Caregiving is a two-way street. The patient needs love and strength and patience, and the caregiver needs love and strength and patience too. Not spending full days with Pete gave me some extra free time. This meant some time for caregiver self-care.

A caregiver must continue doing the things she enjoyed before the illness. For me, that meant continuing to swim with my good friends and my coach on a regular basis. It meant continuing with my Italian classes and my book club. It meant welcoming invitations for lunches with friends. It meant enjoying a glass of wine before dinner and going to bed early. It meant haunting the library and reading as much as I could.

Taking care of myself also meant walking and snuggling with Bella. Bella was—and continues to be—the best self-care therapy for me, the caregiver. She is always glad to see me when I come home. She loves nestling her warm muzzle on my hip, knee or shoulder when I read in bed. Undoubtedly she builds up my ego unnecessarily, but she was the biggest plus factor in my struggles with caregiver stress.

The key is to do the things that will support you in such stressful times. These palliatives will serve as balm to the woes of being a caregiver.

The Long Distance

Keeping a steady rhythm—breathing, stretching, reaching—was something I had internalized from swimming. As I felt the love of my life slipping away from me, I tried to put that rhythm to use. If Pete couldn't maintain his full command of love, I would double or triple the love I had for him. This love would serve us both. I breathed love into both of us.

~13~
PETE'S FINAL LAPS

Memories can be so sweet.

Sometimes in the early evening Pete would say "Let's go down to the beach for a quick dip before dinner." He would put on his faithful Speedo, throw a towel around his shoulders, and we would head west. Our home is only half a block from the ocean. Feeling the water curl over our toes as we walked slowly into the surf never ceased to be invigorating. We stayed close to shore, avoiding big waves, but the cool water was soothing. Pete liked to lie on his back in the water and look up at the sun, and then try a bit of bodysurfing as we headed in to shore. The damp crunchy sand mirrored his big feet as we walked back up to our towels on the beach. After a warm shower at home he always felt ready for a quiet and simple dinner, looking out the window at our fruitful lemon tree.

Time goes on and things change. In December 2014, the last lap of Pete's "swim" began, and on March 4, 2015, Pete passed away.

FOUR FALLS

Starting in December Pete's health deteriorated rapidly. Within a week's time, Pete took four trips to the nearby emergency room. Each trip was caused by a minor fall, when he would try to get out of bed or stand up on his own, especially at night. From one such fall he suffered a hairline fracture of his humerus. It became clear that he could not stand or walk unassisted.

Becoming wheelchair-bound accelerated his physical decline. I had previously gotten a transport wheelchair for him, to take him out for walks in the nearby park, but now he needed a larger and more comfortable chair, for use all the time. How small, stooped, and slouched he looked, with the waistband of his jeans hiked up nearly to his now thin chest. The urge I felt was to scoop him up, lean him on my chest, rock him, and soothe him as I had done with my babies when they were tiny.

He could no longer stay in his room by himself, but needed to be stationed in the common room at the end of his hall, with other non-ambulatory patients. He had difficulty with managing eating utensils, so taking him downstairs to the dining room for meals was more of a challenge. He slept most of the day, with his head falling down to his chest as he sat in the wheelchair. Occasionally I could arrange for him to nap in his room on his bed, but this could only be done with extra constraints and a bed alarm attached to his clothing.

At this point, my emotions were at "High Danger Alert" level. I had prepared myself—or at least hoped I had—to be able to say goodbye. But I soon realized that I had no idea how to control the fear and sadness that were overwhelming me.

I was often tired, but I asked myself how much more tired Pete must be. "You can do this," I repeated over and over to myself.

WHEELCHAIR BOUND

I was saddened but grateful, looking back on the first fifteen months of his stay at the care center, when he was able to do so much more. Just a few weeks prior to his falls, in this same park, he had been able to stand up from his wheelchair and throw a Frisbee for visiting grandchildren. "What a super Frisbee-tosser you are!" I had exclaimed with delight! You can't give enough praise to an LBD patient. It buoys them. But now, praise was not enough

Before long we needed to restrict him from walking at all, night or day. He did keep asking his attendants to let him try to walk. When one finally agreed to get him up and stabilized on the walker, he only made it as far as the hallway before his body melted and he crumpled to the floor. The attendant—who was much smaller than Pete— positioned herself on the floor so that his large body would slump down gradually onto her. Thus neither of them was injured. It was clear that he should not be allowed to try to walk again. We added bed rails to his bed alarm, and rearranged his room so his bed was in a corner, with a wall on two sides

This big change in mobility ushered in other issues. He needed more nighttime monitoring and supervision. These needs caused further financial stretches, because we needed to pay hourly for a special attendant to be in his room with him from 10 pm to 6 am every night. Future expenses looked daunting.

PETE IS STILL THERE

Pete's friend Irish Flynn still came by almost every afternoon. He would push Pete's wheelchair around the nearby park. Pete suggested to Irish that he, Pete, push the chair for a while and Irish could ride in it instead. He didn't want Irish to do all the work. This was classic Pete!

His swim friends arranged a picnic in the park. We pushed him there in his wheelchair, and while he napped through much of it, when he was alert, his smile told us how touched he was. This was the last time he would see some of these friends.

There were still many flashes of Pete's warm and loving insight. One afternoon when I thanked him for marrying me, his response was a swift "My pleasure, ma'am!" Just like out of an old John Wayne movie. That made my day!

Even though the window of what I could do to maximize his quality of life was narrowing, I pushed it open as far as humanly possible. I brought him his favorite flowers for our twentieth wedding anniversary. I told him funny stories. I continued to read newspaper articles and book sections to him. I played his favorite music. And every chance I got I would sit next to him, so I could put my arm around him and we could feel each other's warm closeness.

When he had trouble expressing himself in words, I found that asking him to "talk around it" was useful. And of course, since we were two kindred souls and I knew him so well and loved him so much, I could often surmise or deduce what he wanted to say.

I wondered what he was feeling deep inside? How would I myself feel, no longer being able to direct or control my body?" And the very foreboding question of how close he was to dying pushed itself in. To answer these questions, I turned to love. Some days I had to dip deep into our love reservoir, just as I had sometimes had to dig deep to finish a long distance swim race. "Do the best you can," I told myself, "You can do it."

CARING FOR THE CAREGIVER

When the disease progresses to this point, the caregivers must be sure to continue to take care of themselves. Caregivers need nourishment and replenishment.

I continued my daily activities and connections with friends. I made a concentrated effort to keep up my swimming, my Italian conversation group, my music and theater matinees with my sister Judy, and listening to CD courses. I walked and snuggled with Bella. I took a brief trip to Colorado to visit children and grandchildren, knowing that Pete was in good hands. I couldn't have been as strong as Pete needed me to be if I hadn't set some priorities for my own care.

Even though there were many days when I worried that Pete's death was close, I also realized that no one knows when that time will come – and it could very well be months or years. I could create a "caregiver's trap" if I expected too much of myself. I knew he was well cared for at the care center, and I had built a foundation for him there–one in which he felt comfortable and his professional caregivers had grown to love and look out for him.

LAST GOODBYES

In being so close to the situation, the caregiver has often mentally played out several scenarios for their loved one's passing, so the actual onset of the end-of-life brings few surprises. Perhaps the lengthy preparation eases the overwhelming sadness that accompanies the loss.

Katherine, Susan, and I, along with my daughters Amy and Myla, and sons Jim and John, had some frank and supportive talks about what to expect and what would be best for Pete. We knew that he didn't want to continue living for months or years in his weakened state. We talked and read about hospice and agreed that their philosophy about keeping a patient comfortable without resorting to heroic means was wise and compassionate. We researched different hospice organizations, with the help of the care facility staff, and selected a suitable hospice company.

Their representatives came to interview Pete, and to provide a much-needed hospital bed and commode to help the care center staff with Pete's daily needs. He displayed end-of-life symptoms, like not wanting to eat. One's natural inclination is to help (spoon-feeding, cutting food into small bits) but truly, the message that your loved one is giving you is that he is getting ready to die.

Hospice offers many advantages. They supply a nurse, a caregiver (for showering and hygiene), a spiritual consultant should one so desire, a music person, and more. We chose a hospice group that already had several patients at Pete's care facility, so they knew how to interact seamlessly with the existing staff.

As it turned out, we employed hospice for less than two days. Through an error on the part of a new employee who panicked when he could not wake him, Pete was taken to a hospital emergency room. This is not allowed for patients on hospice care, and the retirement center staff was most apologetic. However, because a CAT scan was done we found out that Pete had pulmonary emboli at the tops of his lungs.

The emergency room physician said she could dissolve Pete's emboli by giving him heparin, but this was not compatible with hospice. So Pete was returned to the retirement center later that evening and died by early evening the next day. His death was peaceful and painless. I was with him in the late afternoon. He held my hand tightly, stroked my hair and smiled, though he couldn't talk.

I just wanted to be near him, to talk to him, to put the cell phone up to his ear so he could hear family members telling him how much they loved him.

Physical presence was everything. Touch was central. I know in my heart of hearts that he knew I was there and that I would always love him. I told him it was safe for him to go, to embark on that final leg of his journey. "You can do this," I whispered to him.

~14~
CELEBRATING PETE'S LIFE

Shortly after his death, his daughters and I arranged a celebration of his life at one of the nearby beaches. He would have loved it!

The late morning sun warmed and highlighted the pristine bay. Children were playing nearby and sailors were busy readying their boats for sailing. Navy ships and small pleasure craft shared the blue waters of the bay behind the tent where we held the festivities. And they were FESTIVE!

Years ago Pete had written out what he wanted to have happen in case of his death. He wanted people to tell "Pete Stories," and to embellish them, because he knew that any story worth telling was worth embellishing.

Pete had been involved in many groups and activities throughout his life, so it was not a complete surprise when we had to move the celebration to a larger venue to accommodate everyone. Navy men and women, the judges, clerks, and lawyers, fellow swimmers, family, and friends all attended.

Irish Flynn spoke of Pete's self-sacrificing bravery and compassion. Bill Pate, who had been close to Pete for many years, spoke of Pete's judicial career and his love for his family. Our swim coach told lighthearted stories about the pool's "big guy," as the coach always referred to him. Katherine and Susan spoke movingly about their father. Amy, Myla, Jim, and John sat with me and held my hand, their very presence both embracing me and holding me up.

In the receiving line, one of our friends, held my hand and asked "What can I do to make the world a better place, as Pete has done?" To this day, that question touches me deeply.

Several months later we held a second ceremony at the UCSD swimming pool, dedicating a memorial plaque in lane 2, his special place. Two more wonderful celebrations, for the scattering of Pete's ashes at sea, filled my heart to bursting. Both ceremonies were organized by the SEAL team, one formal and one informal, reminding all of us that Pete would forever be a SEAL.

Pete was a remarkable man, deserving of all the ceremonies and kind words spoken about him. One of my lasting memories will be of him teary-eyed, when I passed on a comment from another former judge, Betsy Kutzner, who had also worked in the juvenile court. She had commented on his extraordinary capacity for caring about children—their needs, their emotional capacities, and their individual personalities. I told him exactly what she had said, and his eyes welled up with tears, thanking her for saying such sage things about him. She had, in this simple comment, zeroed in on the very things most important to him: children, families, justice, and love. I treasure that she said it, that he heard it, and that I, as his wife and caregiver, got to be the messenger.

~ ~ ~

At his memorials, most people talked about Pete in terms of his life before the LBD, and I certainly cherish that Pete. As his caregiver, I have to say that I also cherish the Pete I took care of through LBD. For one thing, the man I loved, the core Pete, was always there. His courage and fortitude in dealing with LBD is something I marvel at. Even at the most challenging times, I was so proud of Pete.

I still receive thanks and praise from our friends, and when I hear them say "You brought him through this so beautifully," my heart swims with plenitude. Caregiving builds love, and that is what Pete and I did together. I am proud of this. Going the distance with him on his journey, although painful, was a supreme honor for me.

~15~
A FINAL NOTE
FOR LBD CAREGIVERS

Caregiving stretches the limits of your love. It is filled with sleeplessness and heartaches. It is tough – some days as tough a task as anything you have ever done.

The most difficult part for me was not the physical caring for Pete, but the fact that his vital and engaged life was slipping away. I could not stop myself from forecasting ahead, and knowing that I would be without him mentally, and eventually, physically. This stark reality hits you at the point of diagnosis. From there, you have to move forward, for months or years, despite the reality of that last marker, and instead, pay attention to all the ways you can improve your loved one's life on any given day.

AFTER

After Pete passed, I knew things could not go back to "normal." After all, Pete is no longer here. There are also other things that changed. For one thing, if you have been the caregiver, you have changed, and you will have to spend some time getting to know the new you.

Some of the changes are good. For instance, I learned to deal with new challenges on many fronts. I also became quite skilled at making something positive out of any situation. Another post-caregiving factor is that I am proud of myself. I don't mean this in a boasting way. It is just the simple fact that when I was faced with the challenge of helping Pete through his LBD, I answered that challenge with love. I am proud of the love.

On the other hand, I was tired.

Truth be told, I, like many other caregivers, paid less attention to my own wellbeing than to Pete's. Throughout the book, I have advocated for caregivers to take care of themselves. I will also say that no matter how much self-care you practiced, there has been a toll on you—mentally, emotionally, and physically.

Sweet Sleep

Although I continued activities important to me even while Pete was ill, I wasn't sleeping well. I would awaken after a few hours and find it difficult to go back to sleep. I talked with Dr. Speckart who prescribed some sleep aids, which I used for a while. I gradually weaned myself away from those medications because I didn't like the groggy feeling they caused. I favored natural sleep aids, mostly focusing on what they call "sleep hygiene."

I understood my sleeplessness when I was taking care of Pete at home, but once he moved into the care center I thought sleep would return for me. It did not. When Pete passed, I thought I would regain my ability to sleep soundly. Initially, I did not.

Additionally, I sometimes found myself having symptoms similar to those that Pete had had—forgetfulness, not remembering the reason I came into a room, forgetting dates and times, and the like. I couldn't help but think that maybe what had happened to Pete was now happening to me.

Once when I was driving on the highway I noticed a billboard that said, "Drain clogged? Call us at…" My first read of it was "BRAIN clogged?"—and I laughed to myself.

I soon realized that I don't suffer from LBD. The symptoms I have from sleeplessness are not progressively worsening. I just needed time to unclog my caregiver stress, and regain my former levels of acuity and inner peace. Caregivers need recovery time, because caregiving is draining. Be good to yourself. You can do it!

~AFTERWORD~
THE LONG DISTANCE SWIM

For me, swimming is all about beauty and flow. There is an ecstasy to feeling your body gliding through the water, and a profound joy in feeling the water's embrace. Being in the water is like being in heaven, and the long distance swim is like a five-star vacation there.

I still rise early, for my 7:30 A.M. swim practices and hear Pete calling me Mrs. Sloth. I swim in his lane at the pool, and each stroke is in his honor. When I swim in the ocean, Pete is there, with every breath and every glide I take through those wild and wonderful waves. He is there holding me, smiling at me, loving me.

Pete and I will swim together forever—the distance will be long, and the love will be infinite.

ABOUT THE AUTHOR

If left to her own devices, Betsy's biography would read: Betsy lives with her dog Bella in a 100-year-old house in Coronado.

As her writing coach, I am taking over this space because I felt it was important to add a few facts about Betsy Jordan:

With degrees from Wellesley (B.A. Art History), Harvard (M.A. Art History), and University of California, San Diego (Ph.D. English Literature), she was a full-time Humanities professor at UCSD for 15 years.

Betsy Jordan is a record-breaking, award-winning, master-level swimmer, and she exemplifies the values of Masters Swimming: fairness, fun, and fellowship. In her 40+ years of masters swimming competition, Betsy has set over 40 world records and many national and local records, including All-Star and All-American awards. In 2005 she was inducted into the International Masters Swimming Hall of Fame. You will still find Betsy at the morning swim workouts at UCSD and at the La Jolla Cove on many Saturday mornings.

Pete and Betsy have eleven grandchildren, all of them athletically inclined, some following Betsy into masters swimming competitions.

And just so you know, Betsy met Pete at the swimming pool, and one of their favorite swims was when they swam the Maui Channel (10 miles) together in 2004.

For more information about Pete:
www.peteriddlecelebration.blogspot.com/

~~~

Betsy Jordan is available as a speaker about caregiving and/or Lewy Body Dementia.

betsytjordan@gmail.com
www.goingthedistance-betsyjordan.com

51753217R00091

Made in the USA
San Bernardino, CA
31 July 2017